HOW MEMORY WORKS

How Memory Works—
and How to Make It
Work for You

Robert Madigan, PhD

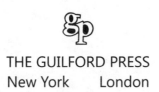

THE GUILFORD PRESS
New York   London

The information in this volume is not intended as a substitute for consultation with healthcare professionals. Each individual's health concerns should be evaluated by a qualified professional.

Printed in the United States of America

This book is printed on acid-free paper.

Last digit is print number: 9   8   7   6   5   4   3   2   1

Library of Congress Cataloging-in-Publication Data

Madigan, Robert.
    How memory works—and how to make it work for you / Robert Madigan.
        pages   cm
    Includes bibliographical references and index.
    ISBN 978-1-4625-2037-4 (paperback) — ISBN 978-1-4625-2038-1 (hardcover)
    1. Mnemonics. 2. Memory.   I. Title.
    BF385.M26 2015
    153.1′4—dc23
                                                        2015007441

To Jodi, for your support all these many years

Acknowledgments

This book was a long time coming, and it would never have made it without the patient support of my wife, Jodi. She tolerated my being at the computer for long periods, and she was the first reader of much of the book. Many of its illustrations profited from her ideas and refinements. My good friend and former colleague Dick Bruce was another stalwart, always ready to look at yet another draft. I owe special thanks to Jo Ann Miller, the editor who helped me discover the book I really wanted to write and whose suggestions and input made every chapter better. Kivalina Grove improved several of the drawings. The folks at The Guilford Press were always helpful and easy to work with, especially Kitty Moore, Chris Benton, and Carolyn Graham. And finally, I thank the students from my memory classes for feedback on the various memory techniques, feedback that led to improvements and new applications. I offer them my best wishes for their futures.

Contents

Introduction

The Art and Science of Memory

Have you ever wished you could better remember the names of people you just met? Or that tasks like paying the phone bill wouldn't so easily slip your mind? Can you imagine going to the supermarket without carrying a list? Or remembering the passwords for all your accounts? Do you wish you could recall more details of the great vacation you took last fall? It turns out that better memory in situations like these is within reach of most people if they practice the strategies of the memory arts.

In recent years science has made great strides in expanding our understanding of how memory works and how we can make it work better. In the pages that follow, you will read about fascinating new research that sheds light on the many facets of human memory. And you will learn about what I call the "memory arts," strategies based on science but applied creatively to handle situations—like recalling a past event or remembering people's names—where forgetting is likely.

You might ask why a book about memory improvement is needed in the age of Google, smartphones, and social media, when so much is literally at our fingertips. It's true that these revolutionary inventions have created a capacity for managing information unimaginable just a decade ago. Interestingly, though, the very power of technology has made improving our memory unexpectedly relevant and valuable. As we outsource more and more mentally challenging tasks to our electronic helpers, we can be left with a sense that important skills are eroding, a feeling that we are getting mentally out of shape. Here is Dan Rookwood, a columnist on style and men's health, writing in *GQ* magazine in 2011:

I used to have all my vital statistics committed to memory—bank account details, passport number, fake date of birth in case I got ID'd. So what changed? I have become over-reliant on artificial memory, that's what. When I wake up, the first thing I do is check my electronic diary to see what appointments I have. When I get into my car, I tap the destination into the GPS—I'd be lost without it. My writing is over-reliant on a computer spell check; mental arithmetic has given way to the calculator. I don't need to remember ye olde postal addresses when my webmail remembers everyone's email for me.

Rookwood is not alone. A survey of 3,000 Britons found that a third of those under thirty could not remember their own phone number, and their memory for family birthdays was far worse. In fact, it would be surprising if this were not the case. Remembering information and appointments requires mental effort, and when a device will easily retain such information for us, why should we bother? Recall how dishwashers and clothes washers, power saws and gas-driven lawn mowers changed how much physical activity we got each day. There was a time when we didn't have to go to the gym to work out. But once labor-saving machines began to take over, we walked less, lifted less, moved less.

Twenty-first-century technology has its impact on mental tasks, not physical labor. Computerized devices and clever software allow us to do more intellectual work than we ever could without them and to do it faster and with relative ease. Whether you are a businessperson using an electronic spreadsheet, a scholar searching through massive databases, a physician relying on computerized records, or a writer dependent on your word processor, most of us would not want to go back to twentieth-century ways.

Indeed, these inventions have become our partners in mentally demanding activities. We count on them to take care of details, sequence tasks, and summarize information. We are so closely partnered with our devices that we become uncomfortable when we must drive to an address without the GPS, or write a letter without the computer, or calculate our taxes without specialized software. That's when, like Rookwood, we start to wonder if something has gone out of balance.

The memory arts offer a way to reclaim some of this lost ground, to improve memory for specific material—remembering facts, numbers, names, events, and more. These strategies rely on initiative, ingenuity, and knowledge of memory principles to make easily forgotten material more memorable, and they do it without outside help. Using them is not unlike seeking out physical activity by deliberately walking rather than driving or taking the stairs rather than the elevator.

Sometimes memory strategies don't require much. If you are introduced to Brad, a new coworker, and want to remember his name, you could picture the actor Brad Pitt standing next to the new Brad, arm in arm. This brings into play two powerful memory aids, visualization and association. In the process, you activate high-level mental processes as you select a mnemonic approach, generate imagery, and create an association. Because this mental exercise is solely under your control and uses only your own mental resources, it is a counterbalance to dependency on computerized devices.

Memory strategies are more than mental exercise. They are practical, proven ways to improve our ability to retain and make use of valuable information. They help in situations where technological devices are least useful for managing information, situations such as remembering Brad's name, remembering to pick up the dry cleaning on your way home, remembering facts for a business meeting, or retaining crucial passwords and PIN numbers. The mental effort and creativity they require is paid back by their usefulness in handling the demands of daily life.

Memory Arts in Action

How much can you improve your memory performance by using specialized techniques? To see what's possible, consider the story of Scott Hagwood. His life was upended in 1999, at age thirty-six, when he received a cancer diagnosis. After surgery to remove the tumor, his doctors recommended radiation but warned that his treatment and recovery would be accompanied by cognitive confusion and memory problems. The news was discouraging to Hagwood because he believed his memory was mediocre at best. He described himself as someone who had graduated low in his high school class and achieved SAT scores barely adequate for admission to college.

Wandering through a bookstore in the days before radiation started, Hagwood bought a book on memory improvement by British memory trainer Tony Buzan. He became intrigued with a method for remembering the order of a deck of playing cards, a method similar to one I discuss in Chapter 14, "The Memory Palace." He tried the technique and got to the point where he could reliably repeat the cards in order after looking at them only once. At a family event, he demonstrated his new prowess to his brother, memorizing a deck of cards in ten minutes and winning a bet in the process.

For those who have never seen it, the feat of reeling off fifty-two cards from memory is stunning to watch. Hagwood's brother was amazed. He wanted to know more. Hagwood told his brother about the U.S. Memory Championship, an annual event where people compete on the basis of speed and accuracy to remember a variety of materials, including a deck of cards. His brother, now brimming with enthusiasm, pressed Hagwood to participate in the 2001 competition. Slowly the idea took root. To compete, he would need to excel in memory for five kinds of material: playing cards, names and faces, poetry, random numbers, and word lists. He searched out memory techniques and began a training program. By the time of the competition, he was ready.

When the scores were tallied, Hagwood was declared the overall Grand Champion of the match. He won again in 2002, 2003, and 2004, the last year he competed. His performance in 2003 set a U.S. record when he memorized 107 random words in fifteen minutes and recalled them in order with correct spelling. It was a record that stood until 2011, when Sophia Hu beat it by memorizing 120 words in the same amount of time.

In 2003 Hagwood took on another memory challenge by meeting the requirements for an international award known as the Grandmaster of Memory offered by a London-based group. To achieve this honor he had to memorize 1,000 random digits in an hour, ten decks of cards in an hour, and one deck of cards in less than two minutes. He met all these requirements, and Scott Hagwood, who had once worried about his memory, became a certified memory whiz at age forty-one.

Hagwood's remarkable pursuit of memory expertise was a personal quest. Few people aspire to be memory competitors, and this is not a book about training for such an endeavor. Rather, Hagwood's story illustrates how powerful memory techniques can be when they are coupled with practice and effort. In the following chapters you will see how you can apply the kinds of strategies Hagwood used to improve your memory in everyday life.

The Science of Memory

The techniques described in the book come from many sources. Some are from contemporary researchers who study memory. Some are from skilled mnemonists like Scott Hagwood. Some have been in use for centuries, going back to Greek and Roman times. In fact, many powerful mnemonic techniques originated in the eras when written works were in short supply and students were taught without textbooks, a time when memory skill was admired and cultivated. But regardless of the origin of the techniques, they can be understood today in a richer way than at any previous point in history because we can now draw on the modern science of memory. Western ideas about memory have changed radically in the last fifty years. Specialties like cognitive psychology and neuroscience have brought fresh methods to the study of the mind, with computerized testing, brain scans, and sophisticated statistical analyses. Surprising discoveries have emerged about different kinds of memory, about the way the attention system operates, how short-term memory works, how memories are recalled, to name just a few. It is not an overstatement to say we are in the midst of a Golden Age for the study of the mind. And in this work, the study of memory has been central.

This new knowledge has much to offer anyone interested in improving memory. Research has demonstrated the superiority of certain memory techniques, like visual imagery, and studies have clarified how best to make use of them. New ways have been found to improve memory in common situations, such as remembering to carry out tasks or retaining facts over time. Scientific advances have provided better ways to analyze why forgetting occurs and what mnemonic strategy can best improve retention. I have drawn on these developments throughout.

The Book

This book is based on my experience teaching memory classes in college and community settings for more than three decades as a professor of psychology at the University of Alaska Anchorage. I've found that people are able to apply different techniques most effectively when they understand the fundamentals of the memory system. Knowing how memory works is the best way to make it work for you. So that is the focus of the first part of the book. You'll learn about the different kinds of memory, how attention can aid or impair memory, how best to strengthen easily forgettable memories, and how memories are recalled.

In the second part, you'll learn how to apply the techniques you've learned to specific situations—including remembering names, appointments, facts, numbers, shopping lists, future intentions, and performance skills. My goal is to help you improve your ability to retain information without help from smartphones, electronic tablets, or sticky notes.

One lesson I learned from working with the methods myself and teaching them to others was that the only way to master memory enhancement techniques is to use them. It is one thing to understand a recipe; it is quite another to cook a tasty dish. This realization led to one of the key features of the book: regular opportunities to practice memory techniques.

Here is how it works. At the end of each chapter, I select a key idea and explain how to retain it using a mnemonic technique. I call these sections "The Memory Lab," a place where memory strategies are put to use. Different techniques are featured in each chapter, so every common memory aid gets its day in the Memory Lab. As you try out the various methods, you see how well different memory strategies work under realistic conditions. As a bonus, you also acquire memory aids for remembering important information from the book. It seems fitting that memory techniques be applied to retain information about improving memory.

What you ultimately will get from this book will depend on what you put into studying and practicing the techniques. As with any other skill, there is no shortcut to proficiency. But I am convinced, on the basis of my experience as a teacher and practitioner of the memory arts, that if you do your part you are likely to see real improvement. And along the way you will enjoy the rewards that come from seeing your mental efforts produce practical benefits from a better memory.

PART I

The Basics

1

Four Ways
of Remembering

Our modern understanding of memory began on August 25, 1953, when a reckless neurosurgeon performed a radical operation on a twenty-seven-year-old Connecticut man who suffered from epilepsy. The patient's name, Henry Molaison, wasn't made public until his death fifty-five years later, but his initials, H. M., were known by generations of memory researchers. He is one of the most famous medical patients of all time because the crippling effects of his operation led to revolutionary insights about the nature of human remembering.

H. M.'s epilepsy resulted from a childhood bicycle accident and gradually became worse so that by the time of the surgery he was enduring ten blackouts a week and occasional full seizures. His family doctor referred him to a hospital in Hartford, Connecticut, where he was seen by William Scoville, a well-known neurosurgeon.

Scoville's particular expertise was in lobotomies, a surgery that involved cutting nerve fibers to and from the front of the brain. He had performed more than 300 of these operations on patients with serious psychological disorders like schizophrenia. It is a controversial procedure, one long since abandoned. Although it sometimes calmed agitated patients, it could also leave them zombie-like and unable to carry out normal daily activities. As it happened, Scoville was trying out an alternative to the standard lobotomy when H. M. came under his care.

Scoville believed that surgery on a region of the brain called the limbic system might produce fewer side effects than traditional lobotomy, and he had special interest in a structure called the hippocampus. At the time its function was unclear—possibly something related to emotion or smell.

Based on little more than a guess, Scoville focused on the hippocampus for H. M.'s treatment. Surgical interventions for epilepsy remove or isolate specific brain areas to disrupt the uncontrolled neural signals that cause seizures. Following this approach, Scoville made plans to excise H. M.'s hippocampus. A colleague with experience in treating epilepsy warned Scoville that the operation was unlikely to help and carried significant risk for the patient. Scoville was undeterred.

Removing either of the two hippocampi—there is one on each side of the brain—would not have been disastrous, but inexplicably Scoville elected to excise both, along with surrounding tissue, thereby ensuring that the functions performed by these structures could no longer occur. A disastrous outcome became apparent as soon as H. M. arrived in the recovery room, where he immediately showed severe memory problems. And there was more bad news. The very next day, the seizures began again, although they were not as frequent.

To Scoville's credit, he didn't try to hide his error. He contacted Wilder Penfield, a neurologist renowned for his work on epilepsy, and told him about the operation. At first Penfield was furious, but he realized the important implications the case held for science. He passed word to the psychologist Brenda Milner, a researcher experienced in amnesia. She immediately made arrangements to study H. M.

The results of her tests were unambiguous: H. M. was unable to form new memories. As Milner told a reporter later, "this was an intelligent, kind, amusing man, but he couldn't acquire the slightest new piece of knowledge. He lives today chained to his past, a sort of childlike world. You can say his personal history stopped with the operation." The first detailed description of H. M.'s impairment appeared in a 1957 issue of the *Journal of Neurology, Neurosurgery and Psychiatry*. It provided an astonishing account of H. M.'s handicap.

> This patient's memory defect has persisted without improvement to the present time, and numerous illustrations of its severity could be given. Ten months ago his family moved from their old house to a new one a few blocks away on the same street; he still has not learned the new address, though remembering the old one perfectly, nor can he be trusted to find his way home alone. Moreover, he does not know where objects in continual use are kept; for example, his mother still has to tell him where to find the lawn mower, even though he may have been using it only the day before. She also states that he

will do the same jigsaw puzzles day after day without showing any practice effect and that he will read the same magazines over and over again without finding their contents familiar. This patient has even eaten lunch in front of one of us (B. M.) without being able to name, a mere half-hour later, a single item of food he had eaten; in fact, he could not remember having eaten at all.

Remarkably, though, Milner's careful testing showed that H. M.'s mental functions other than memory were unchanged. His IQ was 112, about the level of a typical college student. His memory for events prior to his surgery was vivid and intact, and he often talked about these earlier times. He showed no difficulties with comprehending abstract ideas, solving reasoning problems, and making arithmetic computations.

In addition, H. M.'s short-term memory—the ability to retain a phone number while dialing it or to remember a thought long enough to express it—was unharmed. This demonstrated to the researchers that the short-term memory system was separate from the one controlled by the hippocampus. His functioning short-term memory allowed H. M. to use language and converse normally except for his profound forgetfulness. It also allowed him, within limits, to be reflective and observant. He knew he had a memory disability due to an operation, and he was aware of the constant challenge to find clues in the environment to guess what was expected of him and what he needed to do next.

Milner's ongoing work with H. M. uncovered another surprising facet of his handicap. In the early 1960s she decided to find out if H. M. could learn new manual skills. She gave him the task of tracing over a geometric figure while he watched his hand in a mirror. This is tricky because the mirror image is left–right reversed, but with practice people learn how to do it. Milner reasoned that any improvement by H. M. would show that he remembered eye–hand motor skills. She gave him several opportunities to trace the figure on three different days.

The graph on the next page shows his progress.

Every day that he worked at this challenge, he improved, and after three days he was doing quite well, tracing the figure more accurately and doing it in much less time. Despite his growing skill, however, H. M. had no conscious memory of ever having done it; each day he approached the task as if he had never laid eyes on it before. His memory for life events was decimated, but his memory for eye–hand coordination was operating normally.

This experiment dramatically revealed the presence of separate

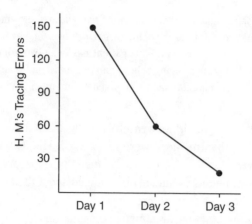

memory systems for different kinds of human experience. The idea was not itself new; psychologists traditionally distinguished between short- and long-term memory. But beyond that there had been no compelling evidence for any other specific form of memory. Now there was.

At first the researchers believed that motor skill was a special case, a complement to a general long-term memory system assumed to store all other kinds of past experiences. However, as research efforts pressed on, study by study, decade by decade, a different picture emerged, one that now includes several forms of long-term memory that range from major systems visible in daily activities to subtle, esoteric systems handling specialized situations. Four of these systems are important players in the coming chapters, each a distinct form of long-term memory, a distinct way of retaining the past.

H. M.'s surgery affected two of the four memory systems: his "episodic memory," the ability to remember new "episodes" or life events like eating lunch or reading a magazine, and his "semantic memory," the ability to retain new facts about the world like the names of H. M.'s attendants or the layout of his living space.

Remembering Experiences and Remembering Facts

The distinction between these two systems was first made in the 1970s by the eminent memory researcher Endel Tulving; it has since become a foundation for modern views of human memory. Tulving proposed that episodic and semantic memory systems differ from one another not only in the information they retain but also in how we recall it.

In the case of episodic memory, remembering involves traveling back in time and reexperiencing what happened earlier. Think about the dinner you had last night. Can you go back to that time? Were you sitting at a table? What did you eat? Was it tasty? Did you get enough? Did you use a napkin? What happened with the dishes when you were finished? To answer these questions, you must access a specific episodic memory by mentally returning to the scene and finding remnants of the sights, sounds, tastes, and feelings from that time. Notice how readily you were able to retrieve aspects of the dinner as you focused on the table, the dishes, and the food, recapturing different parts of that experience. For Tulving, the sense of returning to an earlier event and reexperiencing it is the defining property of episodic memory, one that distinguishes it from semantic memory, our storehouse of facts.

Now try recalling a semantic memory by saying to yourself the name of the first president of the United States. Do you know the number of pennies in a dollar? The capital of France? The colors of the American flag? These facts probably came instantly to mind, appearing in consciousness more quickly than yesterday's meal. The retrieval was also a very different experience. This impersonal information—not linked to the specific place and time when you acquired it—lacks the sensory richness of episodic memories. Ask adult Americans just exactly how they learned that George Washington was the first president and you get blank looks. It's just something they know. We all have a rich store of semantic memories—facts, concepts, names, terms, and more—potentially useful bits and pieces of knowledge long separated from when and where we encountered them and ready to move into consciousness when needed.

Time Traveling via Memory

It is mental time travel that gives episodic memory a qualitatively different feel from semantic memory. Locating a past experience in time is a sophisticated cognitive achievement. It starts with our sense of time, which itself is an advanced ability. Children are almost school age before they have a solid grasp of the present as a point in time flanked on one side by the past and on the other by the future. But episodic memory requires one more step, an even more impressive mental calculation: the ability to return to a moment in the past and reconstruct it from a personal perspective. This feat is important because it clarifies what in fact does the traveling in mental time travel. It is our sense of self that moves back on a timeline to the desired memory, and we accomplish this without losing the vantage point of the present. When you come across pictures of a trip you took last summer, you may pause for a moment to allow your episodic memory to take you back to the adventures of that time, remembering specific experiences, reliving what you did and felt, what you saw and heard, before returning to the present and going on with the day.

The self is not limited to traveling backward; it can also journey forward to the future. Indeed, in Tulving's view, the episodic memory system is as much about our projecting our imagination into the future as it is about reliving the past. Not only can we remember a previous trip; we can also plan a new one. Planning, anticipating, and daydreaming are similar to recalling, reviewing, and reminiscing. And the two faculties are linked. Children develop the ability to time travel in both directions at the same age, usually around five. Older adults who have trouble remembering recent happenings also have difficulty imagining the future.

Episodic memory is our most sophisticated memory system. Its intricate workings probably explain why it is the last memory system to appear in childhood, the first to decline in old age, and the one most vulnerable to disease, head trauma, and lack of oxygen. The complexity of episodic memory has led scientists to wonder whether other animals also experience it. Tulving believes that this kind of memory is fully developed only in humans and that other animals know the past in a more limited way.

Connecting Facts

The unique value of episodic memory in no way diminishes the contributions of semantic memory, which is our knowledge base, our dictionary, our own private Google. It is more than a storehouse of facts; it also creates connections among them, so that when we recall one fact or concept we also gain access to related information. Semantic memory is thought to start with recent experiences. During sleep, these new episodic memories are "replayed" in a process that both strengthens them and identifies the associations, relationships, and patterns that become semantic knowledge—like the association between George Washington and the first presidency. But that's not the end of it. A newly discovered fact is also linked to related information in our network of knowledge. Once you retrieve "George Washington," you can immediately access other facts you learned about him at different times. You know he was the American general in the Revolutionary War, the young boy who couldn't lie about the cherry tree, and the face on the dollar bill. This is the great contribution of semantic memory. It's not only about facts; it's also about connections among them.

Explicit Memory

When we speak of "memory," it is episodic and semantic memory we usually have in mind. Psychologists call these two ways of remembering "explicit memory" because we readily acknowledge them as memories—both are unmistakably information from the past. Other forms of long-term memory don't really seem like memories even though they are just as much reflections of the past. Consider the act of riding a bicycle. Although it is based on previous learning, it doesn't feel like a memory—it's just something you know how to do. Your body carries out the mechanics automatically as information about how to do it is retrieved and put into play behind the scenes. These skill memories have their roots in your first nervous bike ride, your mastery of turning and stopping, and the hours of practice before you rode well. But when you ride a bike now, you are not aware of remembering anything; you are just doing what comes naturally.

Scientists learn about this kind of memory by observing behavior rather than by asking a person to recount the memory. It was behavioral observation that led to the discovery that H. M. could learn a new motor skill. Such memories are called "implicit" because they are deduced from behavior. As we will see, two forms of implicit memory—skills and habits along with Pavlovian associations—are every bit as crucial in our lives as episodic and semantic memories. The diagram on the next page shows the explicit and implicit memory systems discussed in this chapter.

Implicit Memory: Skills and Habits

Much of what we do each day requires little explicit memory. We tie our shoes, cook, eat, drive, and avoid obstacles with hardly a thought about how we accomplish these tasks. These procedural skills and habits are based on

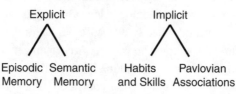

Long-Term Memory

Explicit   Implicit

Episodic Semantic   Habits   Pavlovian
Memory   Memory   and Skills Associations

implicit memories built up over the years and then retrieved at just the right moment. They form slowly through trial and error as successes and failures refine behavior patterns and optimize them for efficiency.

This process was recently brought home to me when I bought a pair of shoes that were slightly longer than my old ones. I discovered how well tuned my stair-climbing movements were after I began stumbling when my toe caught on the stair. Apparently, I had learned to lift my leg no higher than required by my old shoes. But after a little experience, my system adjusted to a higher and safer movement. We see the same process whenever we drive a different car, use a new cell phone, or learn to cook a novel dish.

Because implicit skill memories are distinct from explicit memories, they remain intact in early dementia, which affects primarily episodic and semantic memory. This was evident in Ronald Reagan's struggle with Alzheimer's disease. The fortieth president disclosed his affliction in 1993, and within three years he was severely impaired—he couldn't recall what he had done each day, and he was unable to recognize people he had worked with for years. Despite these serious explicit memory problems, he played golf regularly, dressed himself in suit and tie, and displayed his characteristic gentlemanly behavior. When visitors arrived, he welcomed them warmly even though he didn't know who they were. When he entered an elevator, he would step back and, with a sweeping gesture, allow women to enter first. These well-practiced behavior patterns were still preserved.

Mental Skills

Many important skills are mental. An expert physician readily diagnoses a puzzling illness by drawing on years of practice that have taught her what to look for and what questions to ask. "Book learning" alone doesn't cut it in a practical situation like this. Mental skills like hers are learned through experience just as motor skills are. Experience provides practitioners with something more than facts, something they find hard to put into words, something about the way they approach problems. For example, expert radiologists differ from beginning ones in that they rapidly zero in on abnormalities in an x-ray, passing over normal-appearing parts of the film so that they can devote full attention to clinically significant areas. Similarly, experienced computer programmers have developed an intuitive ability to see solutions to software design problems that beginners must find by working in a linear, step-by-step manner. Successes and failures give experts a deep repertoire of implicit skills and procedures, which they seamlessly combine with explicit factual information. The hallmark of an expert is this amalgam of implicitly "knowing how" and explicitly "knowing that."

Implicit Memory: Pavlovian Associations

Another implicit memory system is the one famously investigated by the Russian physiologist Ivan Pavlov. The drawing on the next page illustrates the best-known psychology experiment of all time in which a bell is paired with food given to a hungry dog. After a few pairings, as everyone knows, the dog begins salivating when it hears the bell, a response implicitly demonstrating the animal's memory for the connection between the bell and the food. This is a primitive memory system found throughout the animal world, even in such biologically distant life forms as ants and clams. It allows creatures large and small to anticipate important events in their environments.

Like motor skills, Pavlovian associations can be acquired even when explicit memory is seriously impaired. An early example was reported in 1911 by the Swiss psychologist Eduarde Claparède. He described the curious case of an amnesic patient who could never remember Claparède from one appointment to the next. Each meeting required that the doctor introduce himself as if they had never met. The patient's memory problems were the result of chronic alcohol abuse, a condition known as Korsakoff's syndrome that can drastically undercut explicit memory. One day, after Claparède went through yet another round of introductions, he placed a pin between his fingers that pricked the patient as he touched her hand. Later,

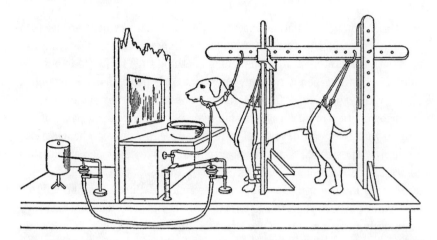

The testing apparatus Pavlov used to discover what came to be called Pavlovian associations.

after she had forgotten that interaction, he reached to touch her hand again, and this time she pulled back. Her memory for the association between the pin prick and his touch was preserved, even though she didn't know why she was leery of his hand.

Pavlovian associations are often earthy, visceral, and primitive, strikingly different from the more factual, intellectual recollections of explicit memory. A person who has been in a serious automobile accident may later react to screeching brakes with a racing heart, sweaty palms, and a surge of adrenaline. These associations are implicit memories retrieved as involuntary, automatic reactions. Because Pavlovian associations normally occur along with explicit memories, the screeching brakes may also bring back the details of the accident as a conscious episodic memory. But in cases like this, it's helpful for us as students of memory to analyze the experience carefully and realize that the gut-level responses represent memory retrieval from a more primitive system. This type of memory was crucial for animals negotiating a complex and dangerous world long before conscious memory evolved, and this ancient memory system continues to play an important role in the lives of advanced creatures like ourselves. We flinch before the doctor inserts the needle, salivate as we study the menu at our favorite restaurant, smile at the sound of a friend's voice, or become apprehensive when we hear a siren. These automatic associations prepare us for important events in the offing.

Multiple Memory Systems: A Major Insight

The discovery of distinct long-term memory systems is a revolutionary scientific advance, one that is the foundation for the modern study of memory. It has allowed researchers to ask more refined questions and discover memory principles unique to the specific types of memory. Scientists now know that episodic memory for new experiences declines slowly over the lifespan, beginning in the thirties, but semantic memory for facts actually improves with age well into the sixties. And the best techniques for developing strong semantic memories are quite different from the best ways to develop good skill memories.

The new perspective has also provided a framework for viewing human memory that is consistent with an evolutionary view of mental abilities. Procedural memory and Pavlovian associations, for example, are based on primitive systems for retaining the past. Both are found throughout the animal world. Explicit memory, on the other hand, is more advanced. It depends on recently evolved neural capabilities and supports sophisticated forms of behavior such as language, reasoning, and problem solving.

The discovery of multiple memory systems helps us understand what it means to be human because it identifies the aspects of the past we are able to retain and use to further our interests. Each memory system captures a different kind of information for a different purpose. Some types of memory are conscious; others are not. Some preserve specific events; others blend them together. Some systems differ little from those found in most animals, while others appear to exist only in advanced creatures, and there is even one memory type that may be ours alone.

In the coming chapters you'll learn more about how these systems work and how to improve them. But long-term memory systems are only part of the picture. The topic of Chapter 2, short-term or "working" memory, allows us to juggle the information we need to deal with the activity of the moment, from expressing a thought to preparing a meal.

 **Introduction to the Memory Lab:
Two Types of Visual Mnemonics**

The Memory Lab section at the end of each chapter gives you a chance to try out different mnemonic techniques. In this first installment I introduce visual mnemonics, which are memory aids based on visual imagery, and illustrate them with a way to remember the four long-term memory systems.

Visual mnemonics are a historically appropriate place to begin learning the memory arts. Ancient mnemonists knew their power and stressed their importance, so much so that most classic mnemonic techniques use visual imagery extensively. Cicero spoke for many ancients when he wrote in 55 B.C., "the keenest of all our senses is the sense of sight, and consequently perceptions received by the ears or from other sources can most easily be remembered if they are conveyed to our minds by the mediation of vision."

The first step in putting Cicero's advice into action is to identify the information needing memory support. I will focus on the diagram on page 16 showing the four memory systems organized as either explicit or implicit. That diagram itself could be enough to help you remember the systems, but I'm going to rework it using more graphic imagery so I can introduce two powerful ways to construct visual mnemonics.

A Mnemonic Based on Direct Visual Associations

The visual image below is a memory aid to help recall the two implicit memory systems. A dog is harnessed in a Pavlovian apparatus and is catching a Frisbee. The Frisbee is a cue for skill and habit memory, and the dog is a cue for Pavlovian associations. If you can remember this image, there is a good chance you can remember the two systems. This

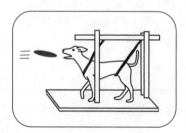

A visual mnemonic for skills and Pavlovian associations based on direct associations.

approach to creating a visual mnemonic is based on finding an image with a direct association to the content you are trying to remember.

A Mnemonic Based on Substitute Words

What about a visual memory aid for the two forms of explicit memory: episodic and semantic memory? Right away we can see a limitation of the direct approach. What possible image could be a cue for "episodic memory"? It's an abstract term, and visual mnemonics use concrete images.

This is a common problem when using visual imagery: not everything we want to remember can be visualized, and so a direct association just isn't always possible. However, there is a workaround, a strategy called the "substitute word technique" and also known as the "keyword mnemonic." It's an approach that has served mnemonists well for centuries. To apply it, we search for a concrete word that *sounds* like the abstract word, and then we create a visual cue for the concrete word. The visual image helps us remember the concrete word, and its sound helps us remember the abstract word. It works like this:

Remember visual image →
    remember concrete word →
        remember abstract word

To apply the strategy here, I chose "exotic salmon" as substitute words for "episodic" and "semantic" memory based on the fact that they sound somewhat similar. Then I created the image shown at the top of the next page. To remember the two explicit memory systems, you imagine the exotic salmon, and the sound of these words helps you remember "episodic" and "semantic."

Using the Mnemonics

I have combined the two images into a single mnemonic also shown on page 22. Take a good look at it because next I am going to ask you to re-create it in your imagination and use it to cue your memory.

When you're ready, close your eyes and retrieve the image. Start by visualizing it from afar so that you can see the full image, with its

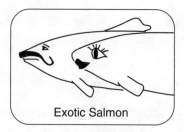

Exotic Salmon

A visual mnemonic for episodic and semantic memory based on substitute words.

two components side by side. Then zoom in on the salmon and mentally inspect it. Recall the substitute words and use them to think of the two explicit memory systems. Give your associations free range so that you can review the characteristics of these two systems. Next, zoom out, move over to the dog image, and repeat the process. If you find your images are fragmented, weak, or fuzzy, that's OK. Just make them as distinct as you can. Expect to see improvements in your mental imagery as you continue to work at it in the coming chapters.

How much memory benefit will this mnemonic provide? That will depend on how well the visual cues work for you and how well you remember the mnemonic. I'll have more to say about both of these requirements in later chapters.

Four Memory Systems

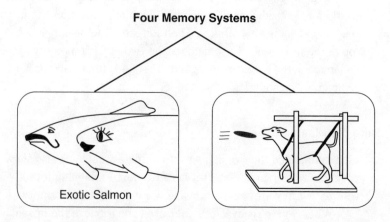

Exotic Salmon

A composite visual mnemonic for the memory systems.

About Visual Images

People differ greatly in how vivid they report their mental images to be. Some describe highly detailed and brightly colored images, but for others, visual images appear washed out, broken up, and fleeting. Fortunately, research has shown that a high level of imagery skill isn't necessary for the visual techniques described in this book. You can expect to receive about as much memory enhancement from weak mental images as from vivid images. Moreover, you can expect your imagery skill to improve with practice. Keep in mind that when you visualize an image mentally you're drawing on the same brain machinery you use in actually seeing something. So the basic equipment is there; it's just a matter of learning to use it. And it's worth doing. Mental imagery not only provides a useful memory tool but is an enriching mental experience, one you may be missing.

2

Working Memory
It's Short-Term Memory and More

To deal with the demands of daily life, we need short-term memory as much as we need the long-term memory systems described in the last chapter. Short-term memory lets you remember what number to press when you listen to one of those long series of telephone options. You rely on it when you're trying to follow the instructions to assemble that new bookcase. Short-term memory holds details we need to get things done. Because short-term memory is so closely tied to accomplishing tasks, psychologists no longer treat it in isolation. They use the term "working memory" to refer to the entire process, both remembering details and carrying out the job. To see working memory in action, follow along with the busy cook in this poem by Jim Daniels. He's got a big order to deal with, and that means juggling information and staying on task.

Short-Order Cook

An average joe comes in
and orders thirty cheeseburgers and thirty fries.

I wait for him to pay before I start cooking.
He pays.
He ain't no average joe.

The grill is just big enough for ten rows of three.
I slap the burgers down
throw two buckets of fries in the deep frier
and they pop pop spit spit . . .
pss . . .

The counter girls laugh.
I concentrate.
It is the crucial point—
they are ready for the cheese:
my fingers shake as I tear off slices
toss them on the burgers/fries done/dump/
refill buckets/burgers ready/flip into buns/
beat that melting cheese/wrap burgers in plastic/
into paper bags/fries done/dump/fill thirty bags/
bring them to the counter/wipe sweat on sleeve
and smile at the counter girls.
I puff my chest out and bellow:
"Thirty cheeseburgers, thirty fries!"
They look at me funny.
I grab a handful of ice, toss it in my mouth
do a little dance and walk back to the grill.
Pressure, responsibility, success,
thirty cheeseburgers, thirty fries.

To serve up that huge order, the poem's protagonist needed short-term memory, focus, and planning. To be sure, memory was a piece of it—memory for the order, memory for the work plan, memory for the status of the meat, the buns, the fries, and the cheese. But just as important were planning, paying close attention, and following through. These functions are carried out in the tightly integrated working memory system that specializes in meeting immediate challenges.

You use working memory when you look up a phone number and keep it in mind while you make the call. Working memory helps you remember "two with mushrooms, one with peppers, and one with anchovies" when you order pizza. It's working memory that makes it possible for you to wander around a store comparing prices of different items and then choosing the best value. It also helps you search the Internet by maintaining your focus and keeping track of what you find. Your success in the search will be determined in part by the ability of the working memory system to keep your purpose firmly in mind and not be distracted by a colorful ad promoting a new movie or a popup offering free financial advice.

Working memory is especially crucial for understanding language because of language's very nature—when you read text or listen to speech, words come to you one at a time. Working memory collects the words and hangs on to them so you can understand the meaning of what you heard or read. When you speak a sentence, working memory is where you gather your thoughts, formulate a statement, and remember the words until you say them. If there is any slippage, you are left in the embarrassing spot of having to admit you forgot what you were planning to say.

The working memory system allows us to make plans, control attention, and carry out actions, all the while providing temporary memory storage for the information we use along the way. One of its hallmarks is flexibility, which is needed because there are many ways to get a job done. Interestingly, that flexibility extends to the different ways people remember information. I see examples of this when I ask students in my memory classes to remember numbers for a few seconds and then write them down. I might show them the number "1081359." Most report that they retain it as speech sounds: "one, oh eight, one, three, five, nine," but some, about ten percent, say they remember it visually, as if they were seeing the number as a mental picture. And occasionally there is an individual who remembers it as the thumb movements it would take to enter it on a cell phone. Clearly, people have options when using working memory.

And these different formats don't exhaust the possibilities. A person can also connect the number with other information and make it easy to remember in that way. One woman saw her mother's birth date (August 13, 1959) in this particular number. So, for her, 1081359 became 10 + 8/13/59, which then became "10 + Mom's birth date." Once she had made that connection, she had no problem remembering it. These examples show that working memory is not a passive repository of information. Each of us plays an active role in how our working memory handles information. What determines the specific format we use might be our personal strengths—visual or verbal talents, for example—or past experiences with similar material.

How Working Memory Works

Researchers believe that working memory results from mental activity at two separate levels. One set of operations are called "executive processes," and they manage how working memory is used. These operations include attention, planning, strategies, and follow-through as we saw with the cook. Executive processes put into action the most advanced parts of the human brain, our highly evolved frontal lobes. The second level of working memory is the memory storage component, where the information is retained and manipulated. It is here that working memory holds on to a number as inner speech or as a mental image or connects it to a fact you know.

The diagram below, based on the work of influential British researcher Alan Baddeley, shows these two levels—executive processes on top and different storage options on the bottom. Two forms of short-term memory, verbal and visual, hold information either in a speech format or as a visual image. There are other types of short-term storage—memory for muscle movements, for example—but the verbal and visual modalities have been studied most, so they are emphasized here. The connection to long-term memory is also important. Even though the working memory system is all about short-term information juggling for the job of the moment, long-term knowledge can be highly relevant, as we saw in the woman who used her mother's birthday to remember a number.

To see how the system operates in the real world, let's return to our short-order cook as he prepares and dishes up thirty cheeseburgers and thirty orders of fries. He probably remembered the order as speech (maybe "thirty and thirty"). Other details were probably remembered visually, such as how many fries remained in the basket, and still others could have been retained as memories of muscle movements, like where he laid down the spatula. He most likely drew on long-term memory for his general work plan, while executive processes managed and sequenced all of this to get the order out.

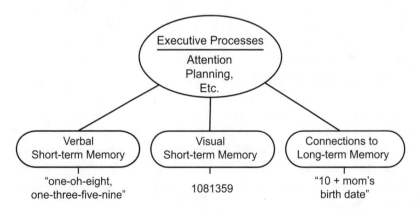

The working memory system.

During this time, his moment-to-moment conscious experience mirrored the operation of his working memory system. When he turned his attention from the grill to the fryer, the bubbling, sizzling fry baskets became the center of his mental world and remained so until he moved his attention back to the grill to see if the meat patties were ready for the cheese. Working memory's operation is believed to determine what we are aware of at any point in time—it appears to be the seat of consciousness.

How Much Can Working Memory Hold?

Working memory has limits. If there is a need to call a number like 1-514-619-4358, most of us will have to look at it more than once to get it dialed. Unlike long-term memory, which is thought to be unlimited, working memory is restricted to a modest amount of information at any one time. Most English-speaking college students can retain seven or eight digits. Remembering a list of grocery items after looking at them once usually has a limit of three or four, and keeping in mind a complex, unfamiliar name, like the Ukrainian city Novomoskovsk, could well be all working memory can handle.

The limit depends not only on the material but also on the person, because people differ in their working memory capacities—differences that turn out to have important ramifications. One way psychologists measure capacity is with a memory task that asks people to listen to a number and then say it backward. So, a person might hear the number "78056" and then recall it as "six, five, oh, eight, seven." This is much more difficult than just repeating the number, and it puts heavy demands on working memory. The test begins by asking a person to repeat two digits backward, and then the number of digits is increased until the person's capacity is found.

Because the backward digit test is often given as part of intelligence tests, there is a large data set available on people's scores. The graph on the facing page was prepared from one such source. Average performance on the backward digit test is shown as the dark, solid line. The two dashed lines above and below that line show the great range of capacity differences people show on the test—ten percent of people have working memory capacities above the top dashed line, while another ten percent are below the bottom line.

The "average" curve shows the differences among people as they age.

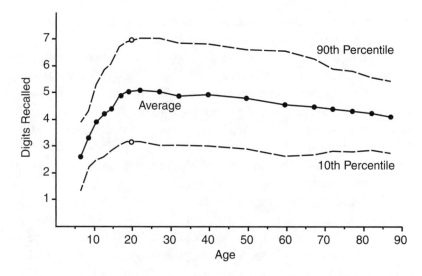

The number of digits that can be recited in backward order as a function of age. Solid circles show the average for all test takers. The two open circles highlight the estimated backward digit memory capacities of twenty-year-olds at the ninetieth and tenth percentiles.

Notice how working memory capacity increases during childhood, reaching a peak in the twenties, and then begins a long, slow decline into the eighties, where it has dropped from a high near five backward digits to about four. Age effects become larger in more difficult memory situations—when handling two tasks at once, for example—but overall, working memory capacity shows only a moderate decline over the lifespan in tests like this one.

It may seem surprising that the decline is not more dramatic given the complaints older people make about short-term memory problems, but the graph shows that the main source of their difficulties is not likely to be memory storage capacity per se. Instead, their problems often come from another feature of working memory, attention. To see how this can happen, consider a person paying bills at her desk who goes to the kitchen for a class of orange juice and then finds herself standing in front of the refrigerator, wondering what she came for. Most likely what went wrong was that her attention was distracted from the orange juice to other topics as she walked toward the kitchen—maybe she saw a plant that needed watering, or maybe she thought about a phone call she needed to make. These conscious thoughts took place in working memory, displacing the orange juice. Once she got to the refrigerator, her purpose had to be recovered. It won't be in working memory because that system was taken over by her wandering thoughts, so she must find it elsewhere. If she is lucky, she will have it in her long-term memory, but if it is not there, she will have to go back to her desk and see if she can think of it again. Once she recalls what she wanted, the orange juice reenters working memory and becomes conscious again. Distracted attention, not working-memory storage capacity, is usually what bedevils older people who struggle with short-term forgetting. We take up attention in the next chapter.

The big story in the graph is not the changes that take place with age; it is the dramatic differences in the capacities of people of the same age shown by the dashed lines. Take a close look at the memory of twenty-year-olds. I have used open circles to show a twenty-year-old at the ninetieth percentile and another at the tenth percentile. There is a huge difference between their memory capacities—more than a factor of two! Variations in memory this large are bound to matter, and they do.

Differences in working memory capacity are related to performance in many situations in which intellectual effort is required. For college students, reading comprehension can be predicted directly from tests of working memory—those who recalled the most details from text passages were the same ones who scored high on working memory capacity. These students were also better able to use context to understand the meaning of unfamiliar words. In tests of reasoning ability, adults with strong working memories were able, on average, to reach correct conclusions more rapidly and more often than others. Students mastering a computer language did so faster if they showed high scores on working memory capacity. In a study of airplane pilots, those with high working memory capacity showed better "situation awareness," which is a pilot's grasp of the terrain around the plane, the location of other aircraft, instrument readings, and flight control settings. The less experienced the pilot, the more important working memory became.

The relationship between working memory capacity and performance has raised questions about its tie to basic intelligence. In fact, studies show a surprisingly tight relationship between working memory and one specific component of IQ, the type required to think logically and solve novel problems. This ability is called "fluid intelligence," and it is measured with test questions such as the one shown on the facing page. The connection to working memory is so strong that there has been speculation that the two

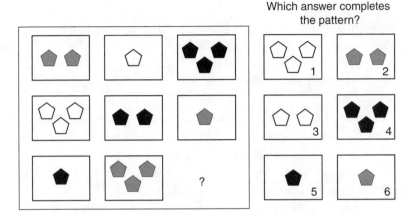

Which answer completes
the pattern?

A typical question from a test of fluid intelligence.

are in fact one. While most researchers say this is going too far, there is without doubt substantial overlap. The available evidence predicts that a person who shines on working memory tests will also be adept at solving problems, acquiring new skills, and scoring well on IQ tests.

Although working memory capacity is important, most of life's routine challenges don't strain it. Like the short-order cook, most of us can manage to plan and organize our efforts to meet our responsibilities. Where working memory capacity matters most is in novel or mentally demanding situations—like a first attempt at cooking a cheese soufflé, with its tricky steps and precise timeline. And even though people with high memory capacity have an easier time in these settings, others also cope successfully. As we accumulate more experience and knowledge, our working memory capacity matters less. In most situations, working memory is more influenced by knowledge, experience, and memory technique than by raw capacity.

Chunking and Organization in Working Memory

When researchers measure working memory capacity in the laboratory, they use unfamiliar tasks like remembering digits backward because the goal is to determine a basic mental ability uncontaminated by past learning. But few daily situations are that unfamiliar, and often we can draw on experience to improve performance. For example, if you were given the phone number 18002753733, you would probably not deal with it as one long eleven-digit number but as four clusters: 1-800-275-3733. Grouping digits is a memory strategy we have learned from experience with phone numbers, social security numbers, and credit card numbers. Known as "chunking," this repackaging of information is a proven way to extend working memory's capacity.

Chunking becomes more powerful when it's bolstered by long-term memory. We saw this in the woman who used her mother's birth date to remember a number. It is a general principle of mnemonics that connecting information you want to remember to other knowledge helps you retain the new information. So, while remembering 1-800-275-3733 is indeed an improvement over 18002753733, a more effective chunking is 1-800-ASK-FRED. Now the eleven digits are reduced to two chunks—"1-800" and "ASK FRED," the first based on our knowledge of toll-free calls and the other based on a meaningful phrase derived from words we know. This technique not only helps us retain the number in working memory, it establishes it in long-term memory as well, and once this happens, we will no longer be dependent on working memory to recall it.

Chunking can be carried out deliberately, like the phone number and the birth date, but it can also occur automatically. When an expert learns something new in his specialty, he effortlessly links it to what he already knows and thus receives a memory boost. Consider an ardent fan watching a baseball game. For him, the action does not occur in a vacuum. His rich knowledge of the game provides many opportunities for chunking by connecting the new information to his existing knowledge. Compared to a baseball novice, the fan has a sizable memory advantage for the game.

David Hambrick and Randall Engle put the memory contributions of expert knowledge to a test by assembling 181 people, ranging in age from eighteen to eighty-six, who had widely varying knowledge of baseball. After assessing the participants' working memory capacity and their knowledge of baseball, the researchers had them listen to several minutes of a simulated baseball broadcast between fictitious teams. Here is an excerpt:

> We're back to the action as Larry Jacoby comes to bat. He has a .300 batting average with <u>100 RBIs</u> on the year. Not bad <u>for a rookie</u>. The shortstop moves into position for a pickoff, and the outfielders swing around to the left. Here comes the pitch—a <u>hard groundball</u> is hit to the <u>left side of the infield</u>. The <u>shortstop</u> dives and stops this one from going into the outfield.

The underlined phrases show information that was later tested. What had the greatest influence on how much the participants remembered? Was it their working memory capacity? Their knowledge of the game? Their age? Hambrick and Engle used statistical techniques to assess the unique contribution of each of these factors to memory performance, and their findings are shown in the bar graph below. It's clear that knowledge of baseball was by far the best predictor of how much they remembered. While working memory capacity and age did matter, their influences paled in comparison to the benefit baseball knowledge provides.

It makes sense that relevant knowledge should play a big role in memory. An experienced fan would know that rookie Jacoby's performance numbers are more than just "not bad"—they are impressive, and so it is no surprise when Jacoby delivers a solid hit. For the fan, Jacoby's rookie status, his performance numbers, and his hit link together into a meaningful chunk. The fan would also understand the nuances of a "pickoff" and probably have a mental image of how the players positioned themselves for it. All of this takes place naturally as the fan's deep knowledge of the game captures and retains the many details, effortlessly connecting new information with stored knowledge.

The fan gets another benefit because the facts and chunks are not only meaningful in themselves but also fit into the overall structure of a game the fan knows well—the innings, the score, the outs, the runs. Each event

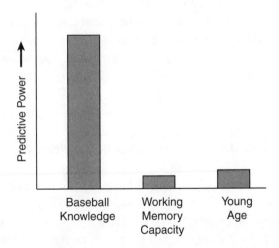

Predictors of the ability to remember information about a baseball game.

plays a role in the familiar drama of a baseball game, and this organizes what was heard into a meaningful story. When it comes time to recall, the fan draws on organization provided by the game itself to access the facts easily. This is an advantage denied to a baseball novice, who must recall isolated bits of information.

Similarly, when master mechanics look under the hood of an ailing car and survey the mass of hoses, wires, and objects, they see a set of familiar systems with sensible interconnections, a perspective that minimizes demands on working memory and frees up mental resources for diagnosing and fixing the problem. This is not the case for fledgling mechanics. Expert cooks understand a complex new recipe on a different level from kitchen beginners, and their working memory for the recipe will be superior. A chess master codes the state of the chessboard at a more sophisticated level than a chess novice, and this better memory leads to better decisions about the next move. In each case, past experience provides a way to reduce the load on working memory and succeed in situations impossible for the novice.

How Many Chunks?

Chunking and organizing improve memory retention in both working memory and long-term memory, but when it comes to working memory, an upper limit is always there, even for the expert. In a definitive analysis, memory researcher Nelson Cowan showed that working memory for adults maxes out at three to five chunks no matter the material. Better packaging of information, as helpful as it is, cannot get around what appears to be a fundamental limit on how much we can keep in consciousness at the same time—typically, four chunks and sometimes fewer. This means that most people can remember the number 1-800-275-3733 but falter at 1-800-275-3733-3283.

The Nature and Nurture of Working Memory

We have seen two sides of working memory. One shows itself in novel circumstances, when we're faced with an unfamiliar problem or when we need to learn a mentally demanding skill. People with high working memory capacities have an advantage in such settings. This aspect of working memory appears to be difficult to change and to some extent may be inherited.

The other side of working memory, the side that benefits from knowledge and experience, is more flexible and can far overshadow the importance of innate capacity in familiar situations. At the heart of these benefits are the operations of chunking and organization, which increase our ability to hold on to information. This frees working memory from a limit set by native ability and moves it to a new limit set by the amount of material that can be packaged into about four chunks.

Memory improvement techniques also rely on chunking and organization to improve retention. We saw an example in the last chapter when I presented the visual mnemonic shown below as a way to help us retain the four long-term memory systems. The memory systems are encoded as two chunks and presented in a visual arrangement that serves to organize them.

Working memory is at the center of the action when creating and using a mnemonic like this. During the creation phase, executive processes decide what kind of memory aid to devise. They supply the planning, imagination, and effort needed to identify the chunks and find images to represent them. The visual and verbal memory areas of working memory are the sites where possible designs are evaluated and refined. When it comes time to use the mnemonic, working memory holds the image while its cues are used to retrieve information from long-term memory.

In the next chapter we examine one of working memory's most important executive processes, attention, the ability to stay focused on a task in the face of distractions. Attention is as essential for the memory arts as it is for remembering in daily life. Although it is no surprise that attention is related to memory, you may be surprised at the ways this relationship comes about.

Four Memory Systems

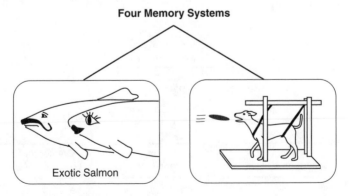

A visual mnemonic for the four memory systems of Chapter 1 encoded as two chunks of information.

In the Memory Lab:
The Picture Superiority Effect

One reason visual imagery has been so popular among mnemonists and memory teachers throughout the ages is that vision is such a strong sense for humans. Our notable visual abilities are directly related to our primate ancestry. Researchers estimate that about fifty percent of the primate cerebral cortex is involved with processing visual information, making vision a sensory system where we have especially good hardware.

A practical application of our visual strengths is what psychologists call the "picture superiority effect." Just changing memory information from a verbal format to a visual format can often aid memory. In a typical demonstration, people are given lists of words to study such as necktie, spool, train, pig, and needle—all concrete words—and they try to retain them for a period of time. Sometimes the lists are presented as printed words, other times as pictures. The consistent finding is that people remember the lists better when they see them as pictures.

In this visit to the Memory Lab, I invite you to try out this advantage by remembering the theory of working memory presented in the chapter in a more visual format. First, look at the diagram below—it is the one I presented earlier with all essential information given as words. The picture superiority effect says that it would be easier to remember if it were more pictorial.

A visual version appears on the next page, where icons represent

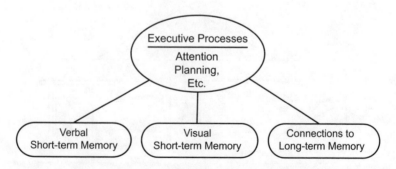

The working memory system represented by words.

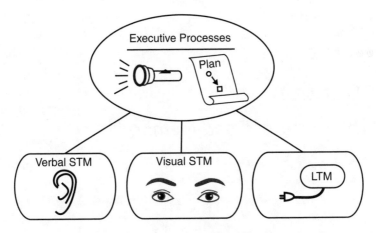

The working memory system represented as pictures.

key aspects of the theory. A flashlight represents attention, and a diagram represents a plan. The ear, eyes, and a plug to make connections to long-term memory depict the three storage options in the theory. But there is an important caveat about this new diagram: I chose these particular icons to represent the theory because they work for me. To give the picture superiority effect a fair test, it's important that the icons be meaningful to you so that when you recall them you'll know what they refer to. If you find that any of my icons don't work, feel free to substitute your own.

Using the Pictorial Version

To give this diagram a try as a memory aid for the theory, you'll first have to firmly establish it in your memory system. The best way is to practice recalling it. After giving the new diagram a good look, close your eyes and recall it. Start by visualizing it from a distance so you can mentally see the whole design without focusing on specific details. Then zoom in on the different parts and recall what they refer to in the theory.

You can check how well this works by testing your memory for the theory after a few days. To make this memory aid longer lasting, you will likely need to practice it multiple times. We'll get into how best to do that in later chapters.

3

Attention

"The Secret of Good Memory"

On an August evening in 1967, David Margetts, a violinist with UCLA's Roth String Quartet, finished rehearsing several Beethoven pieces at about 10:00 P.M. and headed out to his car for the trip home. He carried with him a treasured instrument worth about $800,000, an eighteenth-century Stradivarius violin that had been donated to the UCLA Department of Music. On the way home, Margetts stopped at a convenience store for milk and orange juice before driving on to Gus's Barbeque in South Pasadena for a snack. It was when he got back to his Corvair some fifteen minutes later that he noticed the violin wasn't there. He panicked.

Part of his distress was that he wasn't certain it had ever been in the car in the first place. "The hours immediately following the disappearance I wasn't sure," he later said. "You think of all kinds of things." At 12:40 A.M., when he filed the police report, he noted that it was most likely that he had left the violin on the car's roof.

But after Margetts thought about it more, he came to believe that he had put the violin in the car. "I remember setting the objects down so I could unlock the door," he testified later. "I remember putting in my briefcase, the single fiddle case behind the seat, the music stand, and then putting the Strad in the car." The difference between the two versions of what might have happened is significant, because it is the difference between a theft and a random fall from a moving car. The theft would have occurred at the convenience store, since that was the only place he left the Corvair unlocked. If the violin had fallen off the top of the car, it would have likely happened as he headed out of the parking lot. But to Margetts's dismay, he had no clear recollection of whether or not he had actually placed the violin in the car or rested it on top while he loaded the other items. The crucial action had failed to leave behind a usable memory.

Margetts and UCLA both did everything in their power to get the instrument back. Ads were placed in newspapers, notices were sent to pawn shops and musical instrument stores, the police and the FBI were contacted. But for twenty-seven years the violin remained lost. Then, one day in 1994, a violin teacher brought a student's instrument into a store that specialized in violin restoration. The shop's owners quickly recognized that the violin was special and possibly a genuine Stradivarius. Many of the surviving Stradivarius violins have been photographed and cataloged, and so it was with this one; it was known as the "Duke of Alcantara," after an early owner. Once the instrument was identified, it was a short step to the discovery that it was the violin that had gone missing from UCLA nearly three decades earlier.

It turned out that the student had been given the violin by her ex-husband, who had received it from his aunt, a retired Spanish teacher who played the violin. As the aunt lay dying in 1979, she had retrieved the violin from under her bed and given it to her nephew, telling him that she had found it beside a freeway on-ramp. After prolonged negotiations and a cash settlement, the Stradivarius was returned to UCLA, where it remains today.

The question for us is why was it so hard for Margetts to recall whether or not he had put the Stradivarius in the car on that August night. Certainly he remembered many other details—where he went, what he bought, whether he locked the car, where he parked. Yet when it came to what he did with an object he valued deeply, his memory was a blur.

The most likely explanation for Margetts's memory lapse involves the subject of this chapter—attention. Those aspects of his trip that he attended to created serviceable memories he could access later, but aspects of the trip that took place when his attention was distracted led to weak and unreliable memories. And his attention could easily have slipped when he was loading his car, a familiar, almost automatic activity. He could have been thinking of other things. Would he be able to correct the rough spots in the rehearsal in time for the performance? Should he stop for gas or wait till the morning? We can't know, of course, but anything that moves attention away from an activity will affect how well we remember it.

You see this when you can't remember where you put your keys, or whether you turned off the stove, or if you took your medication. Although we commonly say, "I forgot where I left my keys," forgetting is a misnomer because there was nothing to forget. A viable memory wasn't formed in the first place because you weren't paying attention when the action happened.

A connection between attention and memory is not news. At the end of the nineteenth century, Tryon Edwards, the author of the popular *The Dictionary of Thoughts*, put it this way: "The secret of a good memory is attention." Since then, research has shed new light on the way attention works, and the emerging picture is not as simple as Edwards thought. One important discovery is that there are different types of attention, each with its own effect on memory. The form of attention Edwards had in mind is now called "top-down attention." Many of Margetts's actions that night required it—going to the convenience store, deciding not to lock the car, driving to Gus's Barbeque. None of these situations was sufficiently routine to be accomplished by an unthinking habit. Each required executive actions, a conscious goal, and top-down attention, the necessary conditions for creating explicit memories. Had Margetts needed to rearrange the stuff in his back seat before he could load the violin, his memory would not have been compromised. With no well-oiled habit to fall back on, he would have had to use the executive processes of working memory to create a plan and carry out the shuffling necessary to make room for the instrument. This would have involved deliberate attention and led to usable memories for the events that transpired.

Thus the best way to avoid getting into Margetts's predicament is to find a way to bring top-down attention into the picture. This could be as simple as deliberately saying to yourself "keys on table" when you put down your keys or wagging a finger at the burners after you turn the stove off or repositioning a medication container after you take a pill. The idea is to make at least one step in your routine a conscious, deliberate act and thus activate top-down attention and strengthen the memory.

Top-down attention benefits both working memory and long-term memory, but the connection between working memory and attention is particularly close because top-down attention is its very foundation. Information enters working memory when it receives top-down attention, and the amount of information your working memory can hold is determined by your ability to keep your attention focused. You are reminded of this when you stop on the road to ask directions. If the directions are at all complicated, you had better stay focused on what you hear or the instructions will slip away.

Cognitive researchers Randall Engle, Michael Kane, and their colleagues provided some of the best evidence for the connection between attention and working memory. They knew that college students differed among themselves in working memory capacity, and they designed a study to see how closely this was related to the students' ability to control attention. One of their attention tests is shown below. The students watched a mark in the middle of a computer screen until a symbol began to flash to the left or right of the mark. The students' job was to move their eyes immediately to the *opposite* side of the screen—that is, they had to look away from the flashing symbol. This is not easy because the eye is naturally drawn to a flashing object, and it takes firm control over attention to look in the other direction. On the surface, this doesn't seem to have much to do with working memory, but if attention is its very foundation, then the students' ability to control their gaze should predict how they did on memory tests. And it did. Those who were better at controlling their attention also had higher working memory capacities.

Why should this be? What exactly is the connection between control of attention and working memory? The accepted explanation is that attention is necessary to prevent distractions from consuming working memory resources. When people with good attention control are given a test of working memory—remembering digits backward, for example—their superior attention skills allow them to stay focused on the digits, reserving all their memory capacity for the test material. As a result, they do well. But when attention control is weak, irrelevant material such as a noise in the room or a random thought can enter working memory and reduce its capacity for remembering digits. Now the result is a lower score on the test. A large body of research supports the idea that the amount of useful material that can be held in working memory comes down to the ability to keep attention focused so that its limited capacity can be reserved exclusively for relevant material.

The Attention Control Task

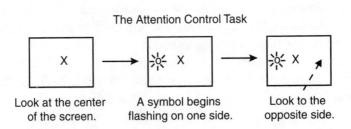

| Look at the center of the screen. | A symbol begins flashing on one side. | Look to the opposite side. |

To get a better idea of what this entails, picture yourself at Starbucks, sipping a latte and reading a novel. If other patrons are talking among themselves and music is playing in the background, your attention can wander. Should it momentarily drift to the conversation at the next table, the snippet of talk you hear enters your working memory, consuming some of its limited capacity, displacing words from the novel, and you find yourself needing to reread the sentence. Making the best use of your working memory is a matter of staying focused.

Top-down attention is also required to create new long-term memories for events and facts. But the role it plays in long-term memory is different from the one it plays in working memory because attention is only the price of admission to the long-term system. Other factors determine how robust the new memory will be—including the importance of the memory, the emotion associated with it, and how frequently you use it. You pay attention to most of your daily activities—what you ate today, what you wore yesterday, what your spouse said to you as you left the house—so they are initially registered in your long-term system, but they are forgotten in the following days because they were isolated, inconsequential events. Attention doesn't guarantee a new memory will endure, but without top-down attention, it won't be there at all.

The Other Forms of Attention

The top-down network isn't the only form of attention—other attention networks also affect how we focus on our world. These rival networks can compete with the top-down network and can disrupt the memory operations it supports. Before we examine these interlopers, keep in mind that it would be disastrous if the top-down system were our only way to direct attention. To appreciate this, go back in time for a moment and imagine a predator moving in on one of our prehistoric ancestors as he is picking berries. He is doomed to become the creature's lunch unless some odd noise or shadowy movement unlocks his attention from the berries and redirects it to the threat. And that's where bottom-up attention comes into the picture. A suspicious sound detected by the bottom-up system will immediately disrupt berry picking and refocus the picker's mental resources on the danger he faces.

The two forms of attention evolved together to satisfy distinct purposes. On the one hand, attention must lock in on the task of the moment—like picking enough berries for a midday meal. But it also must switch focus instantly if anything untoward happens, like the appearance of a dangerous animal. This is a tricky balance. If top-down attention is disrupted too easily, our ancestor would be scattered and ineffective, but if bottom-up attention is too weak, he could wind up being the creature's next meal. The attention system is the result of evolutionary fine-tuning to balance these twin demands.

Advertisers know that the bottom-up system specializes in pulling you away from whatever you are doing at the moment. Those ads that pop up on the margins of the article you're reading on your screen have an impressive record of drawing attention away from the task at hand. This approach is taken to extremes in settings like the Las Vegas Strip, where the words and pictures on signs dance about, change color, and make noise to create irresistible attention magnets. We don't decide to pay attention; attention happens.

It is the intrusive nature of bottom-up attention that leads to memory problems. As you are being introduced to a guest at a party, someone's laugh off to the side pulls your attention away, and later you discover you can't remember the guest's name. Unexpected bottom-up events can be potent distractions that undermine the creation of new memories by interfering with the top-down attention they require. If a child cries or a phone rings as you are trying to follow the soup recipe, you might have to go back to the cookbook to refresh your memory. I will have suggestions for dealing with distraction in a few pages, but first you need to know about a third attention network that has only recently been discovered.

The third network is neurologically distinct from the other two and responsible for a completely different form of attention, one that also has the potential to derail top-down efforts. This network is not directed at the outside world but is focused inward instead. You experience it when you are lost in thought, oblivious to what's going on around you. Scientists call it the "default-mode network," and it controls attention when we aren't focused on the world outside our bodies. It is active when we daydream, when we fret over our problems, when we plan what we are going to do, when we reminisce about the past. It is active when we are in our own inner world. The diagram on the next page shows how the default-mode network occupies a place as one of three distinct attention systems. It plays a special role in our mental activity by filling in when our cognitive machinery would

Top-Down Network
Goal-Directed Attention
"The Secret of a
Good Memory"

Bottom-Up Network
Stimulus-Driven Attention
An ouside event
directs attention

Default-Mode Network
Attention Turned Inward
Daydreaming,
worrying, musing

The Three Modes of Attention

otherwise be idle. If the outside world doesn't hold our attention, this specialized network kicks in and turns our attention inward.

Sometimes the default mode is associated with useful purposes, as when we think through a problem or make plans for the future, but often the network free-associates and simply produces daydreams or loosely coupled thoughts. We all know the detached look of someone who is "not there"—someone who has mentally drifted away, a person whose inner thoughts have trumped the outside world. At that point, the default-mode network is running the show.

The default mode can be every bit as distracting for top-down activities as an intruding bottom-up event. Have you ever caught your thoughts wandering while you're reading a magazine article to the point where you have no idea what the last sentence said? Researcher Jonathan Smallwood calls this type of attention lapse "zoning out," and most readers know it from first-hand experience. What happens is that the default mode takes charge and brings meaningful reading to a halt. Zoning out even shows up in readers' eye movements. In one study, research participants were fitted with eye-tracking devices to record exactly what word they focused on at each moment during a reading session. Periodically, the researchers interrupted the readers to ask whether they were zoned out or fully focused at that moment. When participants reported they had been focused on reading, their eye movements right before the interruption showed uneven progress across the page, speeding up over certain words and slowing down for others. This is a characteristic of normal reading: we take more time to read less common words—"ascertain," for example—and move quickly over familiar words like "accepted." But when readers were zoned out, their eyes moved at a more even rate regardless of the word, a sign they had stopped extracting meaning from what they saw and were just going through the motions of reading.

Zoning out not only affects memory for the specifics of what you read during the zone-out; it also degrades your overall understanding of the text. This occurs because reading requires us to pull bits and pieces of information together into an overall narrative. The more zoning out, the more impoverished our understanding becomes for the larger meaning of the work as well as its specifics.

Zoning out shows how attention can shift between top-down processes and the default mode. It is one example of the ongoing competition among the three attention networks to determine the focus of our conscious experience from moment to moment. This competition can be palpable in busy settings when you struggle to stay focused on a conversation with a friend or the work in front of you. Will attention be controlled by the top-down network? The bottom-up network? The default mode? The rules of the contest are simple. Only one network can prevail at a time, and the winner gets to inhibit the losers. The outcome determines how you deal with your world, as well as what you remember and what you forget.

Distracting Situations

When it comes to establishing new memories, top-down attention is the key player. The successes and failures of memory operations often come down to whether the top-down network was able to best its two rivals and prevent their distractions. Just as attention is the secret to good memory, avoiding distraction is the secret to good attention. Unfortunately, this is sometimes a lot easier said than done. Here are common circumstances that test your ability to stay focused.

Highly Practiced Activities

This was what gave Margetts trouble and led to the misplaced Stradivarius. Whenever actions become automatic, top-down attention is optional, and this creates an opening for your thoughts to wander as the default mode takes control. Once that happens, memory slippage is a real possibility.

Multitasking

This defining feature of modern life makes especially severe demands on top-down attention. You are talking on the phone to a client when the beep of the computer draws your attention to the screen; without interrupting your conversation, you attempt to formulate a response to the email, at the same time keeping your eye on the clock so you won't miss the afternoon meeting, which is starting in fifteen minutes. There is no practical way to avoid multitasking these days. But it runs up against a fundamental bottleneck in our cognitive apparatus, because you can only give top-down attention to one pursuit at a time. As you juggle the phone, the email, and the clock, you have to mentally switch between them. When the email is the focus, attention to the phone conversation must be put on hold until attention can be moved back to it. With each switch, inefficiencies and slippages threaten both your performance and what you remember. You may miss a key detail from the phone call, forget your train of thought when responding to the email, or ignore the clock and be late to the meeting.

The most immediate consequence of an attention switch in multitasking is that working memory is disrupted. As your attention moves from the phone to the screen, memory for words of the conversation fades as the email content becomes the focus of working memory. When you switch back to the phone call, conversation details must be reestablished, and this is where problems can develop. Researchers have found that restoring working memory after a task switch is sometimes incomplete, setting the stage for memory failures. Older adults are especially vulnerable to these working memory problems, although all ages are affected. Even at its best, multitasking is less efficient than performing one task at a time.

Anxiety-Based Distraction

Let's say an important event is coming up—a speech, an exam, a job interview, a first date—and you're worried about your performance. You've got butterflies in your stomach. But the anxiety isn't usually the biggest danger; it's what comes next that causes real trouble. That's when anxiety revs up the default-mode network and turns your attention inward. Consider the test-anxious student. As the exam sits on his desk, his attention is taken over by a stream of anxious thoughts:

"I feel I don't know anything—what's wrong with me?"
"If I fail this test, I've blown my grade."
"Nobody else seems to be having trouble with the test."

As the student frets about his situation, his working memory is occupied by his anxious thoughts, not the exam. Instead of applying his full cognitive ability to the test, he diverts his resources to ruminating about his distress. If the default network is allowed to prevail, his worst fears could well come true. And if that happens, he may believe that his memory failed him, but his real problem was derailed top-down attention.

Weak Motivation for the Goal

Top-down attention is all about keeping mental assets focused on the goal of the moment. When motivation is intense and the goal is clear, attention is strong, razor sharp, and effortless. We all experience situations where we are so engrossed in what we are doing that nothing else matters; at times like these the other networks simply can't break through and distraction is not a problem. But when motivation is weak, it doesn't take much to overwhelm top-down attention—a passing thought or a noise in the room can readily turn attention in a new direction. Maintaining attention when you are poorly motivated requires deliberate, willful effort to stay on task. It can happen to the teacher grading student essays or the worker trapped in boring but socially required small talk with a boss. Both are vulnerable to wandering attention, with memory lapses that could lead to embarrassing *faux pas*. Unless motivation can be pumped up, it will be a continuous battle against distraction.

Staying Focused

Can anything be done about distractions? While there is no simple secret to keeping top-down attention on target, there are strategies that can help.

When Threatened with Distractions, Try Talking to Yourself

Athletes and coaches are well aware of this strategy. Athletes are not only vulnerable to outside distractions that can trip the bottom-up system; they are also subject to worries, insecurities, and concerns that can trigger the default mode. Either way, their top-down attention suffers and their performance is affected. Self-talk—"Keep your eye on the ball," or "Work your kick," or "I can do this"—keeps their attention focused and their motivation strong. There is no magic formula as long as the self-talk is positive and focused on the goal of the moment. Even simple statements like "just do it" or a question like "Am I going to do this or not?" can put you on the right track. Self-talk has also been shown to help test-anxious students stay focused on the test, and it is applicable to other situations as diverse as avoiding mind-wandering during a conversation, ignoring roadside distractions while driving, and resisting the urge to surf the Internet while responding to emails or writing reports.

When Your Attention Flags, Try Tapping into Your Curiosity

We have all struggled to stay attentive during an unexciting lecture or a boring meeting or even at a lackluster dinner party. Low motivation makes top-down attention a struggle. One way to boost your attention is to deliberately create curiosity—which enhances motivation by activating goal-oriented brain structures. Once these areas fire up, top-down attention occurs naturally. Reuben Halleck, a nineteenth-century psychologist, offers this perspective:

> When it is said that attention will not take a firm hold on an uninteresting thing, we must not forget that anyone not shallow and fickle can soon discover something interesting in most objects. Here cultivated minds show their especial superiority, for the attention which they are able to give generally ends in finding a pearl in the most uninteresting oyster. When an object loses interest from one point of view, such minds discover in it new attributes.

Curiosity has another memory benefit besides the top-down attention it promotes. Once your curiosity is satisfied by new information, you have added to what you know about the memory material—a proven way to enhance memorability. So when you ask the person you just met if she spells her name "Vickie" or "Vicki" or "Vicky," not only does your attention zoom in on her name, you pick up an additional fact—the correct spelling—that will help retain it.

When You're Faced with a Tedious Activity, It Can Help to Create a Challenge

One way to improve attention is to make the task more challenging—so challenging that attention naturally occurs because it is required. Psychologist Mihaly Csikszentmihalyi, who has studied these matters extensively, has found that when the challenge is at the right level the task will not only engage attention but also lead to a rewarding experience that produces a state he calls "flow":

> Flow is a subjective state that people report when they are completely involved in something to the point of forgetting time, fatigue, and everything else but the activity itself. . . . The defining feature of flow is intense experiential involvement in moment-to-moment activity. Attention is fully invested in the task at hand, and the person functions at his or her fullest capacity.

The key to creating flow, says Csikszentmihalyi, is to have specific goals that are challenging but attainable and to identify a source of immediate feedback so you can evaluate your performance. Even mundane activities that ordinarily don't hold our interest—wrapping gifts, ironing a shirt—are candidates for the flow experience when the conditions are right. Consider the task of doing laundry: gathering the clothes, sorting the dark colors from the light, putting them into the washing machine, then the dryer, and finally folding and putting them away. To add challenge to this routine, you would work at becoming more efficient (eliminating backtracking and wasted movements), more thorough (leaving no sock behind), and faster (short total time). Feedback comes from observing your progress and timing your efforts. When the challenge is right and flow is achieved, top-down attention becomes easy and memory is improved.

This approach can be applied in situations where memory is the primary objective, such as learning the names of people in a group or mastering the information in a technical article. By setting specific goals and monitoring performance, you create a challenge that turns a low-interest task into an engaging game that not only is less onerous but also produces stronger memories.

For students of memory, attention is a core process, one that not only determines what gets into the memory system, but also, as we will see later, what we retrieve from it. But attention is only the first step in acquiring a strong memory. In the next chapter we explore proven techniques that build on attention for robust, lasting memories.

In the Memory Lab: Designing a Visual Mnemonic

In this installment, we walk through the process of developing a visual mnemonic. The goal is to have a reliable way to remember the three actions you can take to get attention back on track: using self-talk, becoming curious, or creating a challenge.

Find a Visual Cue for Each Action

This is a crucial step. The time you spent finding a good image to cue each of the actions will repay itself every time the mnemonic is used—the more direct the association between the image and the strategy, the better. My choices are shown below. Remember, though, that memory cues are individualistic, so images that work well for me might not work for you. If one or more of them don't provide an obvious association with the strategy, try to come up with something better.

Visual Cues for Attention Strategies

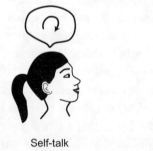

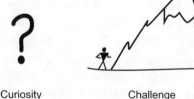

Self-talk	Curiosity	Challenge

Next, Bind the Images

At this point we have helpful visual cues for each of the attention strategies. But we need to consider the possibility that we might forget one or more of the images, which would make the mnemonic useless to us. Retention of the images can be improved if they can be bound together in some way so that they are recalled as a group rather than as three separate images. I have already taken one step in that direction. Look at the way I placed the three images side by side when I introduced them. This created a perceptual grouping by configuring them as a threesome, pulling the images together and making them easier to remember. A perceptual grouping is the most basic way to bind images together.

In the drawing below, the perceptual grouping idea is taken to the next level, with a circle serving as a frame around the images, giving them even more pronounced spatial relationships with each other and therefore stronger binding.

However, a much more powerful way to bind the images is to integrate them into a single meaningful composite, as I've done in the drawing on the next page. It shows a climber carrying questions to the summit and talking to herself. The climber as the main focus of the image serves to chunk the cues into a cohesive image.

These two steps are common in the creation of visual mnemonics:

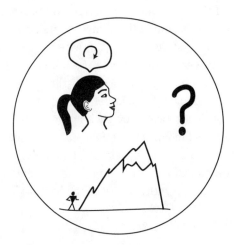

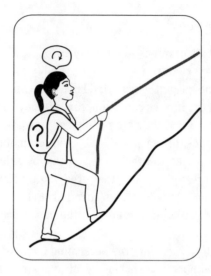

first, find memory cues for the desired information; second, make sure the images will be retrieved together by connecting them in some way. There is still one last step that should be included with any newly fashioned mnemonic, and that is to strengthen it in memory by rehearsing it—mentally visualizing the mnemonic and using it to recall the three strategies. I will have more to say about rehearsal in the next chapter.

Here is one last point about creating visual mnemonics: Don't let them get too complex with too many parts—it increases the chances that some of the cues will be forgotten. My personal rule of thumb is to limit a given image like the climber to a maximum of three or four memory cues. So, what would I do if there were six strategies to retain rather than three? I would create the mnemonic so that there were two separate sections to it, each with three cues. For example, the mnemonic could show the climber followed by a dog on a leash with three memory cues located on each figure. (The leash is to help bind the dog to the climber.) Or I might imagine there is another visual mnemonic in the climber's pack, and I would visualize a portion of it conspicuously sticking out to remind me to mentally look in the pack for a separate image with the rest of the memory cues.

4

How Dragons Make
Strong Memories

People who take my memory classes sometimes ask me to name the best way to strengthen memory. Unfortunately, there's no simple answer because so much depends on the situation. But there is a small set of techniques that are especially powerful and widely applicable. These tried and proven memory principles are what this chapter is about. I call them the "Dragon Principles" because they are represented by a curious acrostic:

Romantic Dragons Eat Vegetables And Prefer Onions.

An acrostic is a sentence in which the first letters of the words are cues for memory material—in this case, the seven principles: **R**etention intention, **D**eep processing, **E**laboration, **V**isualization, **A**ssociation, **P**ractice, and **O**rganization.

This acrostic is odd, to be sure, and you may wonder if you will remember it. Be patient. You will see how the Dragon Principles can make the acrostic easy to hold on to, and once this happens you will have at your fingertips a checklist of seven powerful ways to strengthen your memory.

Retention Intention

When you fail to retain some important bit of information—a name, for example—it is often your own fault because, in truth, you never really tried to remember it. You just took for granted that it would stick. But soon you're faced with that vexing question: "Now, what was her name?"

A retention intention sets the stage for good remembering. It is a conscious commitment to acquire a memory and a plan for holding on to it. When you say to yourself, "Be sure to listen to her name and rehearse it," just before the host introduces you to her sister, you have made a retention intention and taken the first step in deliberate remembering. This step begins to pay off immediately. As soon as you commit to a memory goal, attention locks on to what you want to remember. This is how attention works—it serves the goal of the moment. And the stronger the motivation for the goal, the more laserlike attention becomes and the greater its memory benefits, first registering the information in working memory and then aiding long-term retention. As a result, you will be likely to remember the sister's name during the evening, and the chances are good you'll bring it to mind if you run into the two of them a week later.

A key feature of a retention intention is the plan for holding on to the material. It might be as simple as rehearsing the memory, or it might involve one of the memory strategies described later in this book. Whatever the plan, when you are clear about how you intend to retain the material, it is more likely you will actually carry out the plan, and this can make all the difference between a weak and a strong memory.

As an example, suppose you want to remember several questions to ask the doctor on your next visit. This is the time to formulate a retention intention. Your plan might be to create an acrostic with the first letters of the topics you want to discuss, or maybe you will decide just to run over them in your mind several times before the visit. Yes, it's true that you could put the list of questions in a notebook or on your smartphone and carry it to the doctor's office. A memory helper like that works, but one of the goals of this book is to demonstrate that you can handle situations like these without resorting to external memory aids. For a practitioner of the memory arts, a routine memory demand offers an opportunity to use one's wits and knowledge of memory principles for a practical end; it is a challenge to be met head-on. A retention intention starts this process.

Bear in mind, though, that your retention intention must be a firm commitment, not a passing wish. Motivational intensity very much affects what will come of it: when your retention intention is made properly, the chances of acquiring a healthy new memory shoot up.

*D*eep Processing

In an important study, memory researchers Fergus Craik and Endel Tulving asked college students to answer a question about words that flashed on a computer screen. The students were told that the purpose of the experiment was to measure how fast they could answer the questions, but the real purpose was to see how different kinds of questions affected memory for the words they saw.

The researchers discovered that the kind of questions dramatically affected how well the students remembered the words. The bar graph below shows the result of a surprise recall test given right after the students finished. When the question was about a word's appearance ("Is it in capital letters?"), their memory for the word was poor. When the question was about a word's sound ("Does it rhyme with *weight*?"), memory was better. But the questions that led to the strongest memory were those that asked about a word's meaning ("Can it be used in the sentence 'He met a ___ on the street'?"). When the students were required to access meaning and try to use it, retention took its biggest jump.

Craik and Tulving concluded that the questions about a word's meaning required deeper mental processing and that this depth led to better

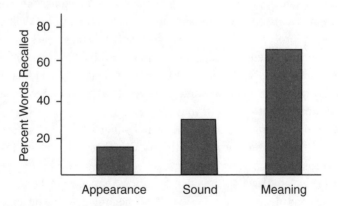

Performance on a surprise memory test after answering different types of questions about words shown on a computer screen.

memory. The other questions required "shallow" processing because they could be answered with surface features of the word—its appearance or sound—without considering what the word actually stood for. Shallow processing left behind weaker memories.

Deep processing is a mental activity that gets at what we know about a topic. The operative word here is "deep," as in deep appreciation, deep understanding, deep meaning, or deep connection. When we interact with memory material on these levels, our efforts produce an enriched memory, one better established and more likely to be retained. Deep processing even shows up in brain scans as increased activity in key brain areas associated with memory. It is this activity that appears to give deep processing its memory advantage.

We constantly move between deep and shallow processing, devoting careful scrutiny to some experiences but sliding over others. Your eyes glaze over as a relative pontificates or an acquaintance rambles. You hope there won't be questions later because your comprehension was so minimal that little remains in your memory. But the reverse is also true. When you encounter something important or meaningful to you, you attend carefully and process it deeply. An audiophile who sees a notice that a favorite group has released a new CD will take in every detail she reads and connect the information to what she knows about the group. As this happens, she is creating a memory likely to survive long after she's forgotten the other happenings of the day.

In this example, deep processing occurred spontaneously because the information resonated with the audiophile. But you can also deliberately activate deep processing as a mnemonic strategy, using top-down control to think about the memory material on a more involved or more detailed or more personal level. So, if you want to retain a health tip you hear on the radio while you're driving to work, you can strengthen memory for it by thinking about how it relates to your life.

Deep processing assumes you can connect the new information with other things you know, and this is not always possible. Take the dragon acrostic, "Romantic Dragons Eat Vegetables And Prefer Onions." This is an isolated fact, a bit of information that doesn't hook up with much else, and deep processing won't be helpful unless you can make some meaningful connections. The next memory principle does exactly that.

Elaboration

It's an interesting paradox that when you add new information to an existing memory, you can actually improve your chances of recalling it. If you choose the information well, it can provide a secure anchor and make the memory more accessible. Elaborating a new memory expands its footprint by better connecting it to your knowledge base. Let's return to our onion-loving dragons to see elaboration in action—but to benefit, you will have to be tolerant of several "facts" you may find questionable.

> *There has been unexpected progress in understanding the flaming breath of dragons. It now appears the flame comes from the combustion of vegetable oil extracted by the dragons' digestive system. This discovery is noteworthy because it explains the strong attraction dragons have to vegetables, especially during mating season. An ample supply of vegetables in a dragon's diet is important to them because a robust flame is necessary for attracting mates—dragons with weak flames are often passed over in the mating process.*
>
> *The new insight also sheds light on dragons' unusual preference for onions. It has long been known that dragons fight over access to wild onions. The study revealed onions play a special role in the dragon flame because their vegetable oil contains trace elements that produce colorful effects when burned. The result is a flame believed to have erotic effects on dragons of the opposite sex.*

This new "knowledge" is added to your memory store and links the dragon acrostic to what you already know about courtship, seduction, and mate competition. Suddenly it becomes clear why Romantic Dragons Eat Vegetables And Prefer Onions. The new information changes the acrostic from a strange statement to a meaningful, even reasonable, observation about the romantic life of dragons. Now the acrostic is much more memorable. Elaboration has added new associations, expanded meaning, and allowed deeper processing.

One of the best ways to elaborate memory of easily forgettable material is to ask the question "Why?" The deeper and more extensive the answer, the better it will work. It doesn't even need to be true, as we saw in my fanciful elaboration of the dragon acrostic. Indeed, when you practice the art of memory, you are free to use your imagination, and fantasy elaborations are completely legitimate if they are helpful. Primal themes like survival, sex, aggression, betrayal, danger, or love can provide memorable elaborations. So, when a coworker asks you at a meeting to forward a report to him the next day, you can improve your chances of remembering to do that by inventing an outrageous, urgent reason he wants it. For instance, you might decide he desperately needs to sell it to a competitor to support his drug habit. Playing this memory game with a dash of mischief will make for a strong memory, and when you send the report, you should give yourself a pat on the back for your cleverness.

Visualization

The ancients' enthusiasm for vision as a memory aid is supported by modern research. There is simply no other sensory system that rivals vision in terms of vast capacity for retaining information, a capacity that has exceeded attempts by scientists to measure it. In one notable effort, Lionel Standing, a British researcher, asked young adults to view 10,000 snapshots of common scenes and situations. Two days later he gave them a recognition test in which the original pictures were mixed in with new pictures they hadn't seen. The participants picked out the original pictures with an accuracy of eighty-three percent, a jaw-dropping performance. But even greater feats have been reported in earlier times. Peter of Ravenna and Francesco Panigarola, Italian memory teachers from the fifteenth and sixteenth centuries, respectively, were each said to have retained over 100,000 images for use in recalling enormous amounts of information. Peter used his images as memory cues to retain a detailed knowledge of civil and canon law. The images were arranged in "memory palaces"—mnemonic aids based on the layout of familiar buildings, such as cathedrals in Peter's case. Specific images were associated with different locations in the cathedral—the altar or the baptismal, for example. When Peter needed a fact, he mentally traveled through the cathedral until he found the cue for it. Francesco used his images in a similar way. (Memory palaces are the topic of Chapter 14.)

The ancients had guidelines for creating effective memory images. The most famous surviving suggestions are from an anonymous Roman teacher in a work called *Rhetorica Ad Herennium,* written in about 85 B.C.:

Now nature herself teaches us what we should do. When we see in everyday life things that are petty, ordinary, and banal, we generally fail to remember them, because the mind is not stirred by anything novel or marvelous. But if we see or hear something that is base, dishonorable, unusual, great, unbelievable, or ridiculous, that we are likely to remember for a long time.

This approach has been endorsed by generations of mnemonists, century after century, right up to the present day. The idea is that images are more effective if they include some combination of bizarre, striking, comical, startling, beautiful, ugly, disfigured, or disgusting features. Sometimes all it takes is a good dose of exaggeration to produce these effects. If you want to remember to get onions, a tomato, and celery at the market, you could imagine a huge pile of onions with a giant tomato and an enormous stalk of celery sticking out of the middle of it. Exaggerating the size of a memory object or imagining there are many, many of them can be a quick, easy way to increase memorability. But it will help even more if the images are dramatic and graphic. Here is the fourteenth-century cleric and teacher of the memory arts Thomas Bradwardine explaining to his pupils how to remember the twelve signs of the Zodiac:

> Suppose someone must memorize the twelve signs of the Zodiac, that is the Ram, the Bull, etc. So he might, if he wished to, make for himself in the front of the first location a very white Ram [Aries] standing up and rearing on his hind feet with golden horns. And he might put a very red Bull [Taurus] to the right of the ram kicking the ram with his rear feet. Standing erect, the ram with his right foot might kick the bull in his large and super swollen testicles, causing a copious effusion of blood. . . . In a similar manner a woman may be placed before the bull as though laboring in birth, and in her uterus as if ripped open from her breast may be figured coming forth two most beautiful Twins [Gemini] playing with a horrible, intensely red Crab [Cancer].

The teacher illustrates how to interlock graphic images and thus create a memorable structure that holds the signs of the Zodiac in order. Modern research shows that such striking images are better retained than mundane ones, especially at longer retention intervals. Just what gives them their memory advantage remains a debate among researchers. Is it because they are bizarre? Distinctive? Unexpected? Novel? Emotional? Humorous? Shocking? Whatever it is, the best way to learn how to create good memory images is to experiment to find what works for you. My advice is to have fun and try to inject some special zing. Wacky is good, as is lewd, naughty, gruesome, disgusting, or politically incorrect. So when I meet my new neighbors, Jerry and Barbara, I might associate them with an image of Jerry Seinfeld grabbing the behind of an indignant Barbra Streisand. If I put a little effort into creating the imagery, I'll remember it. In the future, the neighbors will be pleased when I address them by name—and they'll never need to know the seamy way I do it. The best memory images, a student once observed to me, are ones you would never describe to your mother.

Image Interconnections

Did you notice how Bradwardine created interactions between the different parts of his image? He deliberately depicted the Ram kicking the Bull and the Twins holding the Crab because he knew that anytime an image has separate parts, there is a danger it will fragment in memory, and the parts will not be retrieved together. By creating interactions, he bound them together and avoided this problem.

Here is another example. Let's say I want to buy those three items at the store—celery, onions, and a tomato. Inspired by *Ad Herennium,* I imagine a clown dressed as a vagrant juggling the three objects. While this might work, it could also fail because the three objects are separate and any one could be lost, leaving me remembering the clown and one or two of the items, but not all three. But if I pump up the interaction between the parts by making the clown look surprised, with big onions for eyes, a tomato jammed into his open mouth, and celery growing out of his goofy hat, each object will be bound tightly to the main figure. The result is an integrated memory that I will recall intact.

Color and Movement

The Zodiac images not only depict dramatic, interacting scenes; they also are alive with color and movement. The Ram's horns are golden, and he is kicking the Bull. Bradwardine and other past practitioners of the memory arts who encouraged their students to incorporate color and movement were wise to do so. Colored images are five to ten percent more memorable than images without color. Movement has also been shown to improve retention.

The guidelines I've given for visualization represent the ideal. Often, though, you won't have time to achieve this level of sophistication—the memory setting won't allow it. But it is no disaster if the image is bland or if color and movement are absent, because the visual system is so powerful that any concrete image can bestow a memory benefit. In my experience, the advantage of creating a distinctive image with color and movement is that it requires less memory rehearsal to maintain. A practical approach is to create the best memory image you can and then compensate with additional rehearsal if your image seems lackluster and vulnerable to forgetting.

Association

A winning strategy to retain an easily forgettable fact is to connect it to another memory that is easier to recall. Consider the clown and the shopping list. A clown is a distinctive image, readily retained and easily recalled. By being associated with the clown, the grocery items too become easy to remember. When expert mnemonists describe how they accomplish their feats, it is all about associations. Dominic O'Brien, a legendary memory competitor, lists "the art of association" as one of the most important components of his memory skill. Harry Lorayne, an impressive memory performer, uses his highly practiced ability to form rapid associations to remember individual names in large audiences. "The first thing you notice about Mr. Fleming's face," he explains, "is his large mustache. See it burning, *flaming*. Mustache = Fleming." Joshua Foer, a journalist turned memory competitor, won the 2006 USA Memory Championship in part by memorizing the order of a deck of cards in one minute, forty seconds. He achieved this after spending a year developing his ability to make speedy associations that turn playing cards into memorable images. For example, when the next three cards are the five of clubs, five of spades, and six of diamonds, he has learned to associate them with an image of celebrity Dom DeLuise delivering a karate kick to the groin of Pope Benedict XVI. He mentally puts this image into a memory palace and moves on to encode the next three cards. Later he will return to the memory palace to retrieve the image and recall the cards.

The possibilities for associations are vast. Those we have seen in the Memory Lab were based on vision and language, the stalwarts of the memory arts. Other modalities also affect memory—smells, tastes, and sounds are powerful cues—but they are not easily incorporated into mnemonics. However, there is one modality, emotion, that has strong potential to enrich associations based on vision and language. When emotion is added to an association, it strengthens its memorability. What are the scenes you remember best in a book or movie? Not the casual conversations, but the encounters where emotion is heightened, where feelings reign, where anger or grief or romantic passion are in the foreground. The "base, dishonorable, unusual, great, unbelievable, or ridiculous" images recommended by *Ad Herennium* evoke emotional reactions. If I create my clown image with imaginative gusto, I give it humor and whimsy, qualities that add one more association to the memory and help bring it to mind.

Indeed, in some cases, emotion may determine whether information is recalled at all. Consider Joshua Foer's image of Dom DeLuise delivering that karate kick to the groin of Pope Benedict XVI—this is hardly an emotionally neutral image, especially the way Foer creates it. Later, when he is trying to retrieve it from his memory palace, he may experience a hint of "ouch!"—the emotion associated with the memory—and it could be just the added cue he needs to reconstruct the image and remember the cards.

Practice

This principle is simple: memory can be strengthened by rehearsing or refreshing it. You experience the effects of memory practice every day. It is why your friend's name pops into mind when you see him, why details about your favorite team come flooding back when you see its name in a headline, why you have many job-related facts at the ready when you're at work. You can retrieve these memories easily because you have accessed them over and over, a process that creates robust memories. And this is as it should be—the memories you have used frequently in the past are the memories you are likely to need in the future. Practice has made them strong and placed them at your fingertips.

But what about information that doesn't have the benefit of natural memory practice? The name of the woman you met at yesterday's open house, the recipe you saw demonstrated on the Food Network, the points you intend to make when it is your turn to speak. If you don't rehearse such information you can lose it.

Practice is the least glamorous of the Dragon Principles, but it is a powerful way to strengthen memories of all sorts, and it is indispensable for difficult material you must retain over long time periods. When you are learning to play bridge, you have to rehearse the bidding process if you are to remember what you need to do. When you pick a PIN number for a new account, you had better plan on practicing it if you want to use it without looking all over for it. Practice has been singled out for special emphasis by ancient teachers of the memory arts, by professional mnemonists, and by memory researchers. While other Dragon Principles can reduce the amount of practice needed, only rarely can they eliminate it completely. So, even though you incorporate good elaboration, fine visualization, and exceptional associations, plan on engaging in at least some practice if you want to turn forgettable information into strong and lasting memories.

Although the idea of memory practice is simple, whether or not it works depends on how you carry it out. Early rehearsal is especially important because you can begin to forget new information quickly after you acquire it. Think about how many times an address or phone number has slipped your mind minutes after you hear it. Dominic O'Brien, an eight-time World Memory Champion, recommends mentally practicing challenging information like a difficult name or number several times within the first few minutes. You'll need more practice if you want to retain material for days, weeks, or longer. And your practice will be most effective if you space it out. In fact, for long-term retention, the importance of spaced practice is one of the best established principles in psychology, supported by research going back to the early psychologists of the twentieth century.

The best spacing intervals vary from situation to situation. Remembering an unusual name like Sanna Gormina requires a different rehearsal plan than remembering a dinner meeting for next Wednesday at seven o'clock. You'll need to practice a name like Sanna's right away. And that won't be enough if you want to retain it over time. So, how soon should you practice it again? In the case of Ms. Gormina, the added rehearsal should begin fairly soon. The dinner time, on the other hand, is easier to remember and not as vulnerable, so it could tolerate a longer wait before you rehearse it.

Developing a good sense of how to space memory practice is an intuition a practitioner of the memory arts must learn from experience. That said, professional mnemonists have provided useful guidelines. Dominic O'Brien recommends a "Rule of Five": rehearse the memory after an hour, a day, a week, two weeks, and a month. Other mnemonists offer similar spacing advice. Even though O' Brien's rule is not optimum in all situations, I find it helpful if I don't take it too literally—it provides a concrete example that is easy to remember. Difficult material like a tricky name will require tighter spacing; easy material like the dinner meeting can be approached with a more relaxed schedule.

*O*rganization

When material is organized into a meaningful structure, memorability is much improved. Consider a shopping list of eight items. I observe that three items are frozen foods, two are produce, two are from the bakery, and one is in the dairy section. Once I discover this organization, the list will be easier to remember.

Organization helps memorability in two ways because it involves both a process and a product. Creating an organizational structure requires deep processing, which enhances memory. Once the material is organized, relationships and characteristics that weren't obvious stand out, providing associations and elaborations that strengthen memory. The result can be dramatic. In a now classic study, memory researcher Gordon Bower and his colleagues asked college students to remember a long list of words drawn from eight different categories—minerals, body parts, animals, and the like. The students were given several opportunities to study the list and took a test after each attempt. One group saw the list organized into the categories, while the other was given the words in a random order. The group that understood the organization remembered more after studying the list once than the other group remembered after studying it four times.

Ancient and medieval mnemonists knew the value of organization, and they approached it systematically. First, they broke the material into small but meaningful parts, a step they called "division." Next they arranged the parts into a meaningful structure, a step they called "composition." The high regard early mnemonists had for the process is shown by a fourth-century memory teacher who wrote, "What assists the memory most? Division and composition: for order serves memory powerfully."

When the amount of memory material is large or complex, the processes of division and composition are a real benefit. The division step should yield parts that are succinct and easily retained. How succinct? A medieval rule of thumb was that each part should fit in "a single glance of the mind's eye." A modern restatement is to limit the size of each part to the capacity of working memory. Once that is done, the next step is to compose a structure for the parts.

What about an organization for the Dragon Principles? We already have the acrostic to serve as a memory aid, but if we can create an organization for them, we will have another way to remember them. The first step is to notice that the material is already divided into seven succinct principles, so the "division" step in organization is already done. What's needed now is the "composition" step to put the parts into an organizational structure. Looking at the principles, we note that several overlap. When we add material by *elaboration*, we also create new *associations*. Both of these operations require *deep processing*—as does *organization*. We could group these four principles together under the common characteristic that they *expand the meaning* of memory material, each doing it in its own way.

Next we need a theme for the overall organization. One possibility is that the principles are all different strategies for strengthening memory, and this suggests an organizing theme based on memory *strategies*. A retention intention is about making a plan. Visualization makes use of a sensory strength of primates, and memory practice brings into play the universal memory-strengthening operation of rehearsal. The box below shows the Dragon Principles organized as four mnemonic strategies, with one having

---

**The Dragon Principles
as Strategies**

Activate a Plan
    Retention Intention

Expand Meaning
    Deep Processing
    Elaboration
    Association
    Organization

Involve the Super Sense
    Visualization

Call on Old Faithful
    Memory Practice

four parts. The organization not only improves memorability, but also gives us insight into why the Principles are important.

What's Next?

The Dragon Principles help create strong memories, but sometimes even a well-established memory can elude you at the moment you need it—as when you see a familiar person and can't think of her name or when you can't recall the perfect birthday present you had seen for your partner. Finding and retrieving memories is a process separate from creating and strengthening them. In the next chapter, we learn how the retrieval system works and what to do when it comes up short.

 In the Memory Lab:
A Helper Image for an Acrostic

Acrostics like the Romantic Dragon are useful memory aids. They are especially appropriate when memory material can be represented by a series of keywords—as is the case here. But there is one stumbling block: people sometimes have trouble remembering how the acrostic starts. Once you recall the first word or two, the rest usually comes along. So how do you make sure you will readily remember those crucial first words? In this Memory Lab segment, we create a helper image designed to get the acrostic going.

A useful helper image suggests the first words of an acrostic, as the image on the facing page does by depicting a "romantic dragon." Although the drawing as it is makes a serviceable helper image, it could be made even more effective if it had color and movement. Here I invite you to try adding these enhancements to the heart and the flame in the dragon image. These are the two features that connect most directly to the acrostic by suggesting "romantic" and the benefit of vegetables. Let's pump them up with color and movement.

Start by making the heart above your mental dragon red. If you have trouble visualizing red, look at a red object just before you close your eyes to create the image. Next, apply a color to the flame, and then see if you can add movement by making it shoot out as the dragon

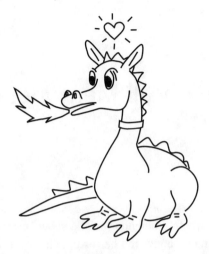

A helper image designed to bring the dragon acrostic to mind quickly.

huffs and puffs. If you have difficulty, it can help to approach movement as animation—a series of still images one after the other. This can get a more natural experience of movement going. Once you get the enhanced image working for you, plan on rehearsing it so that the enhancements bind to the image.

Here is one last thought about these enhancements. Keep in mind that people differ in how vivid their memory images are. If you are someone who has to work to create images, remember that vividness appears to have relatively minor impact on how well images work for memory purposes. If you are able to produce even a hint of color or movement, that's enough for now. Both the vividness of your images and the ease of producing them will improve with practice.

5

How We Recall Memories

Not long ago I ran into a neighbor on the supermarket checkout line. Her ponytail, her runner's body, and her bright blue eyes were familiar, but to my dismay, I couldn't think of her name. We chatted amiably for a few minutes—and I managed to duck the name problem. Not until I drove up to my house some half-hour later did her name come to me. It was Sue, of course.

What exactly was the problem? Sue's name was obviously in my memory system because I recalled it later. So why couldn't I think of it in the supermarket line? It turns out that gaining access to a memory is by no means a sure thing. But as we will see, there are strategies to boost our retrieval skills.

Part of my difficulty was that I don't use Sue's name often; in fact, I hadn't talked to her in several months. So the name memory wasn't all that strong to begin with. Also, I encountered her in a different setting from where I normally see her. Most of us have had this experience: when you spot your dentist at the movies or a former professor at a ball game, it may take a moment to place them. If I'd run into Sue in our neighborhood, there's a better chance her name would have come to me.

Retrieving a memory starts with an appropriate retrieval cue—in my case, that would have ideally been the sight of Sue out in her front yard. An effective cue helps us zero in on one specific memory out of the great store of memories we have available. When a memory is recent or well practiced, almost any cue can pop it out. If I see Sue again soon, I will remember her name, no matter the circumstances. But when a memory is weak from lack of use, a strong, relevant cue is needed to access it. In fact, with the right cue, we can retrieve memories that we thought were long lost. Steven Smith, a cognitive psychologist at Texas A & M University, gives a good example of the value of the right cues. He describes accompanying his father on a visit to Austin, Texas, where the elder Smith had gone to college:

> Having lived most of his life in St. Louis, Missouri, except for two years at the University of Texas at Austin, and four years in the military during the Second World War, my father returned to Texas after 42 long years of forgetting. Although previously certain that he could recall only a few disembodied fragments of his college days, he became increasingly amazed, upon his return, at the freshness and detail of his newly remembered experiences. Strolling along the streets of Austin, my father suddenly stopped and animatedly described the house in which he lived in a location now occupied by a parking lot. He recalled in vivid detail, for example, how an armadillo had climbed up the drainpipe one night and became his pet, and how the woman who had cooked for residents of his house had informed them of the attack on Pearl Harbor, abruptly ending his college career. Not until he returned to the setting in which those long-past events had occurred had my father thought or spoken of them.

These long neglected memories were deeply buried in the father's memory system, inaccessible under ordinary conditions. But when the two men visited Texas, vivid memories poured into the father's consciousness.

You can appreciate the power of memory cues that come from different senses—sights, sounds, smells—when you immediately recognize a picture of the elementary school you attended, or you hear an old friend's voice on the phone, or you sniff a perfume that your mother wore when you were a child. Each situation brings back vivid memories. A friend of mine told me that a mere whiff of chalk could bring forth a flood of images of her fourth-grade classroom.

Even when a cue is potent enough to retrieve some information, it may not bring up all you know about something. Consider my encounter with Sue. At first she registered as vaguely familiar, someone I should know. But at that point I didn't have a clue about who she was or where I knew her from. Once we started to talk, I got more cues and soon recognized her as my neighbor from down the street. But even then the cues were not strong enough to retrieve her name. Memory cues are like that: some are barely able to evoke a sense of familiarity; others can produce a richly detailed memory.

What to Do When Remembering Comes Up Short

Elusive memories can sometimes be activated with specialized retrieval strategies. Here are three useful ways to pry loose a stuck memory.

The "Shotgun" Strategy

Memory retrieval boils down to finding the right cue. But how does one go about that? Memory trainer Tony Buzan recommends temporarily letting go of what you've forgotten and instead turning your attention to what you can remember related to it. This was how I recalled Sue's name. As I drove home, I focused on everything I knew about her—her house, her dog, my opinion of her, the appearance of her yard, her husband's name, Eric. And that's when it came to me. Finally I had it. Life was good.

It pays to explore any and all associations when using the shotgun technique, not only external connections like Sue's house or her husband, but internal ones like my opinion of her or my mood when I last saw her. The goal is to rummage around in your memory until you chance upon a cue that dislodges what you're trying to remember. Of course, some luck is required, but my experience supports Buzan's approach: for me, this technique works more often than it doesn't.

The "Return to the Scene" Strategy

This next method proceeds in a more orderly way than the shotgun technique. The idea is to reestablish the context in which the memory was created. This was what Steven Smith's father did when he revisited Austin. With this technique you can reclaim many stuck memories—recalling your boss's suggestions from yesterday's meeting, remembering where you parked your car, or summoning up what you'd been planning to do before you were distracted. Let's say you leave your desk, head into the kitchen for a glass of orange juice, and suddenly find yourself staring into the fridge with no idea of what you are looking for. Picturing yourself back at your desk and reconstructing what you were doing there just before you left is likely to bring back a memory of the decision to get a cold glass of juice. If this exercise fails, going back to your desk in person so you can experience all the cues directly will usually do the trick.

The "return to the scene" strategy has been researched extensively as a way to interview crime witnesses to obtain detailed, accurate memories. The procedure, called the "cognitive interview," helps witnesses find retrieval cues to bring back useful information. It has been shown to recover about thirty-five percent more information than traditional interviewing.

The officer begins by building rapport so that the witness feels his or her information is important and valued. Next, the interviewer helps the witness reexperience the context of the crime to find cues for retrieval. Sometimes this requires a trip back to the scene, but often the context can be re-created by asking the witness to imagine it. Here is a typical instruction:

> *Try to put yourself back into the same situation as when the crime was committed. Think about where you were standing at the time, what you were thinking about, what you were feeling, and what the room looked like.*

The interview is open-ended, and the witness sets the pace by reporting everything that comes to mind. The interviewer helps out as needed to encourage the witness to try to remember not only crime details but also the contextual cues that might facilitate retrieving them.

The "return to the scene" strategy can save the day when you know the time and place the missing memory was created. Perhaps it's the item you need at the store you thought about yesterday, or maybe it's the great suggestion for your sister's birthday present a friend made, or it could be uncertainty about where on earth the car is parked. When these memories defy other efforts to recall them, it's time to give "return to the scene" a try. Think back to when and where the memory originated. If you can imagine the setting, with its sights and sounds, if you can recall what you were doing at the time and even how you were feeling, you might hit upon the cue you need to rescue that memory.

The "Wait and Try Again" Strategy

Sometimes a name or fact will pop into mind after you've given up trying to remember it—like students who suddenly remember the answer to a test question after they have left the classroom. Unlike the other strategies, the idea here is to take a complete break and attempt to recover the memory later.

Memory researchers Matthew Erdelyi and Jeff Kleinbard conducted an instructive experiment to test the utility of the "wait and try again" strategy. They began by showing people pictures of sixty objects—a watch, a fish, a boomerang, and other random items. They presented the pictures one at a time for five seconds and then asked the participants to recall them. On average, participants could remember slightly more than half the pictures at that point. Then the researchers sent the people on their way and told them to try to remember the pictures three times a day for the next six days. The graph below shows what happened.

With repeated attempts, more pictures came to mind, and by the end of the six days the participants recalled an average of thirty-eight pictures per attempt. In fact, they remembered even more than the graph shows because they didn't bring up exactly the same pictures each time. Sometimes they forgot a picture previously remembered but recalled another picture they had never mentioned before. Over the six days, the participants remembered an average of forty-eight pictures at one time or another. Psychologists call this kind of memory benefit "hypermnesia." Although "wait and try again" works with all kinds of memories, it is especially effective with imagery like the pictures of Erdelyi and Kleinbard. Purely verbal memories, like a name or a word, are helped but not as much.

The strategy aids memory in two ways. When you carry it out, you end up spending more time trying to recall the memory since each attempt adds to the total time you have devoted to remembering that particular item. This can help—sometimes it just takes a while to bring a reluctant memory to mind. The second contribution is the rest periods you take between

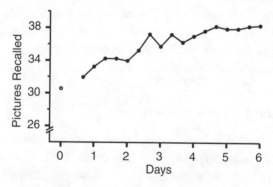

Memory for sixty pictures over six days as research participants made repeated efforts to recall them.

retrieval efforts. They allow you to approach the problem memory anew from a fresh perspective on the next attempt. The research is not clear about just how long to wait before trying again, but a rule of thumb I use is to give it at least ten minutes. During that time, occupy yourself with something completely unrelated.

Of course, not all memories are recallable, even with these strategies. Sometimes the memory itself is just too weak; other times you simply can't find the right cue. But often, with patience, effort, and the appropriate strategy, the memory will come forward. The "shotgun" technique is the place to start, because sometimes it works quickly and it doesn't require much effort. If shotgunning is unsuccessful and the missing memory originated in a specific setting, then the "return to the scene" approach is a good follow-up. And if all else fails, "wait and try again."

Reconstructing Memories

When the memory you're searching for is a fact, like my neighbor's name, you're finished with the retrieval effort as soon as the name pops into mind. But when you're remembering an event, like a business meeting from last week, the memory is more complex. It's like a story with different parts, and it has to be pulled together in a meaningful way. A major insight of modern memory research is that our memories are nothing like a tape recording that you can play back to reveal the event exactly as it happened. It is a much more complex process. To get a feel for it, imagine that you attend a friend's wedding and that night you decide to write about the celebration in your diary.

What do you have to work with? Your episodic memory contains both general and specific information. The general information, called the gist, gives you the main story line—the wedding took place at a resort on the coast; it was a nice affair; the reception was small but fun. The gist provides the big picture and the emotional tone without a lot of detail. You will also retain specifics about the event—the song playing as the bride entered, the purple rose petals scattered on the white runner, the bridesmaids' bouffant dresses, the tipsy groomsmen, the cheesy D.J. As you sit down to write in your diary, you will combine the gist and the specifics to record your impression of the wedding.

Since the wedding memory is so fresh, it won't be hard to retrieve specific fragments—the lace on the wedding dress, how the bride's dad wiped away his tears, the best man's jokes. Each of these details will easily cue others until a narrative emerges. But this kind of unsystematic retrieval would produce a disorganized story. For the purposes of your diary entry, the fragments must be selected, organized, and woven into a coherent account. To do this you will call on high-level processes involving attention, working memory, and executive control to access and organize specific facts and impressions. If you want to describe what the maid-of-honor was wearing, you will deliberately retrieve images of her and her dress. In the end, the memory you recall will not be a replay of the wedding, but a unique creation produced by managing retrieval cues to activate specific details relevant to your developing narrative.

This brings me to the most important point about this thought experiment: the content of a retrieved memory depends on its purpose. If you were to describe the wedding to your parents, it would differ from your diary version. You might stress the décor of the room, or compare the reception to the one at your sister's wedding, or talk about attendees your parents know. The version you relate to your college roommate would also differ. In effect, you would experience a different memory on these retellings. Each account integrates memory fragments into a unique description of the event. The number of fragments needed for these constructions can vary greatly. If your roommate asks, "How was the wedding? Did it come off well?" you might make a summary judgment by recalling only the gist. On the other hand, if your friend wants to know how a former lover behaved at the wedding, you would pull together a more complex and detailed story.

So there is no single "tape" of the wedding. Your experience is stored as a collection of memory details created moment to moment during the event—the exchange of vows, the dancing during the reception, the bride tossing her bouquet, and so on. As memory researcher Morris Moscovitch put it, memory information is just "dumped in and tagged according to elements of its content, to be sorted and organized at retrieval."

Memory Alterations

Every time a memory is recalled, the memory system changes. This happens in part because the process of recalling a memory can itself be remembered, along with when and where the recall took place. You will remember writing about the wedding in your diary along with parts of what you wrote, such as the details you emphasized and the observations and judgments you made. In the future when you think about the wedding, this diary version, or some of it, can come to mind along with other bits and pieces from the event itself.

Interestingly, even the original memory of the wedding can be changed by the act of remembering. Researchers believe that memories briefly enter a malleable phase when they are recalled and become vulnerable to information slipping in or dropping out or changing. Thus the memory system is far from a static archive of past experience—it is dynamic, flexible, and changeable. And this means that completely accurate memories are never guaranteed. The odds of getting it right are best relatively soon after the event, when the specifics are fresh and easily retrieved. But as time passes, details can be forgotten or altered, so you can end up with a good sense of what generally happened but be mistaken on the specifics.

New Zealand researcher Mercedes Sheen and her colleagues offer a fascinating example of this phenomenon. They interviewed twenty pairs of same-sex twins and asked them to recall memories associated with cue words. Following are responses from a pair of identical twins, fifty-four-year-old women, who recalled memories for the cue word "accident":

Twin 1: I remember falling over and really hurting my elbow and knee when a wheel came off my roller skate.

Twin 2: Hang on a minute, are you talking about those roller skates we got for our eighth or ninth birthdays?

Twin 1: Yeah. So what?

Twin 2: Well, that actually happened to me, if you don't mind.

Twin 1: What do you mean? It was me! I was skating with you and . . .

Twin 2: Yeah, with Marie on the old tennis court.

Twin 1: Yeah, but it was me, not you. I remember it being really bumpy with grassy bits in it.

Twin 2: I think you'll find if you really think hard it was me.

Twin 1: Well, I remember it so clearly, and you skated home to get Mum.

Twin 2: No, you skated home to get Mum, because I was hurt and crying and couldn't move.

Twin 1: Oh, well. I guess we get confused; it happened so long ago.

Most of the twin pairs Sheen tested disagreed on at least one memory. Here are other instances: Both thought they were the one who got a nail in his foot. Both thought they were the one who fell off the tractor and sprained a wrist. Both thought they were twelfth in an international cross-country race. Both thought the other one used to grab the dog by its testicles.

Notice how the twins agreed on the gist of what happened but disputed the details. This is the most common form of memory error. Part of the problem comes from the nature of the forgetting process itself—details are forgotten faster than the gist, leaving you with a general sense of what happened but without detailed information about the particulars.

When details are poorly remembered, memory reconstruction draws on all our mental resources, including general information, emotional biases, and reasoning ability, as we try to come up with a recollection that squares with what we think happened. If you try to remember that wedding several years later, you might picture a little girl preceding the bride down the aisle, even though there was no flower girl in the ceremony, simply because formal weddings often unfold this way. It's not that you would deliberately add this detail; it's just that it could seem so reasonable that a flower girl should be there that it would feel true. Attitudes and opinions can influence memory reconstruction, as when you remember a wedding guest whom you have always disliked behaving more boorishly than he actually did. We can even mix up information from two separate events—for example, incorporating details from one wedding into the memory of another.

The most dramatic memory distortions arise when we come to believe in a memory that never happened at all, a memory that is completely false. Elizabeth Loftus, a memory scientist now at the University of California, Irvine, pioneered this line of research by showing how it is possible to plant totally fictitious memories into a person's mind. Loftus began her study by telling the participants, all college students, that she was trying to find out what people are able to remember from childhood. The students gave Loftus and her team permission to interview close relatives to identify childhood events that had happened to them, events that the students would subsequently try to remember. Each student was presented with four incidents, but what they didn't know was that one of them was a complete fabrication, a story about being lost in a mall that relatives confirmed never happened. The bogus story was specific and detailed. It was supposed to have happened to the students at age five in a particular mall where they became lost until found by an elderly woman and reunited with their family. The participants read accounts of the four events and then tried to recall as much as they could about each. Most of the students accurately recalled the true stories, but twenty-five percent of them also "recalled" the bogus event, sometimes in elaborate detail. Other researchers have replicated these findings by inducing research subjects to "remember" phony happenings such as spilling a punch bowl on the parents of the bride at a wedding reception, having to evacuate a grocery store when the sprinkler system activated, and being attacked by a vicious dog. The percentage of participants susceptible to these false memories was similar to that found by Loftus.

In these studies, the false memories occurred when people were given the gist of an event and tried hard to recall the specifics. Eventually they constructed enough plausible details from general knowledge and other memories that the scenario seemed real to them. In fact, when they were debriefed after the study, several participants had a hard time accepting that the events didn't occur.

Memory distortion and false memories underscore just how active the process of remembering is. We don't "roll the tape" when we remember a past event. Instead, we draw on scraps of stored knowledge to fashion an appropriate memory. Occasional errors are a natural consequence of this mode of operation.

Given the possibilities for distortion and error, is there any way to tell whether a memory is accurate? The short answer is that without outside verification there is no way to be sure. We usually have a sense of whether a memory is accurate based on the confidence we have in it—how true and complete it seems as we recall it. Unfortunately, though, memory confidence has been shown to be only a moderate predictor of memory accuracy. Consider the twins' confident but mistaken memories and the college students who were convinced their false memories were true. It is also worth noting there have been more than 200 cases in which DNA evidence has exonerated a wrongly convicted felon who was confidently but mistakenly identified by an eyewitness. This is not to say we should disregard our confidence, but rather that we should be aware that it can fool us.

Another indicator of a memory's accuracy is the amount of particulars it includes. When a memory comes easily and is rich in detail, especially specifics like sights, sounds, or smells, research shows that the memory has a good chance of being accurate. When a memory is vague or when it comes back slowly after effort, the odds of distortion go up. But keep in mind that there is no completely reliable way to tell from the memory itself how correct it really is. The take-home message for all of us is to be a bit humble about the absolute accuracy of our memories and open to the possibility that errors can creep into them.

What's Next?

This chapter completes our overview of the memory system, and we are now in a good position to look at applications of the memory arts. The next chapter gets us off to a good start by looking at two quite different approaches to memory improvement.

In the Memory Lab:
Evaluating and Improving a Visual Mnemonic

Not all visual mnemonics are created equal—some work a lot better than others. In this installment of the Memory Lab, we take a close look at a mnemonic intended to cue the three ways to retrieve a blocked memory discussed in the chapter. The mnemonic would be used in situations where you are struggling to recall a memory and you want to review your options for getting it to come to mind. Here we assess the quality of a proposed visual mnemonic and improve it.

The image on the facing page is a mnemonic for the three strategies—"shotgun approach," "return to the scene," and "wait and try again." The shotgun is a visual cue for the first strategy. I chose the cop to cue the second because of the connection between law enforcement and the "return to the scene" approach. The clock cues the third strategy. Let's see how this mnemonic measures up on three features of a good visual memory aid.

Are the Retrieval Cues Effective?

Cueing the desired memory is the bottom line for any mnemonic. It is entirely possible to remember a mnemonic but not be able to remember what it stands for. The shotgun, the cop, and the clock would likely work for me, although you will have to judge for yourself whether they would work for you. If a cue in a mnemonic turns out to be weak, it is

A mnemonic for three strategies used to recall blocked memories.

not necessarily a fatal flaw, as long as you take steps to strengthen it. Various Dragon Principles, such as practice, deep processing, association, or elaboration, can be brought into play to pump up the cue's effectiveness. An alternative, of course, is to look for a more effective cue.

Are the Image Components Tied Together?

As we saw in the last chapter, when a visual mnemonic has several components—the shotgun, the cop, the clock—one or more of them can be missing when you recall the image. What happens is the image becomes fragmented and components drop out. The remedy is to bind the parts to each other by creating meaningful interactions between them. The cop's hands do this by holding the shotgun and pointing to the clock, but there could be a problem here. The connection between the clock and the cop doesn't really make much sense because there doesn't seem to be any reason the cop would be pointing to it. It is an odd gesture that could be forgotten, and once that happens, the clock could disappear as well.

Is the Image Memorable?

A mnemonic is useless if you can't recall it when you need it. It's annoying to find that you forgot a mnemonic that you created specifically to help you remember something else. My cop mnemonic gets a mixed score on this point as well. In truth, it's bland, and that makes it potentially forgettable. This is a case where memory practice along the lines of the Rule of Five will be required to be able to remember it well.

One way to improve its memorability is to add some action. A redesign of the mnemonic appears below. In this version, the cop has had it with his unreliable clock, and he is blasting it with his shotgun. The new image adds a little violence along with the action, which is always good for memorability. As an extra bonus, the three parts of the image are now bound together more tightly than in the previous version, making forgetting less likely. Memory practice is still called for, but the amount of practice required most likely will be less.

It's worth giving any new mnemonic a quick check with a dispassionate eye to see whether it looks like it will be effective when it is called on in the future. Sometimes, as in this case, there are practical ways to improve it.

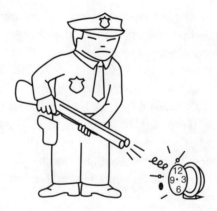

An improved mnemonic for three memory recall strategies.

PART II

Memory Applications

6

Paths to Better Memory

Cicero, the great Roman lawyer and statesman of the first century B.C., had an abiding interest in memory. At a time when the teleprompter was beyond imagining, he delivered elegant, compelling speeches without aid of any kind. Memory, he wrote, is the foundation of the orator's art.

In Cicero's time, memory skill was noticed and admired. For him and his contemporaries, memory took two forms, and the distinction between them is central to this chapter. One was called "natural memory." It's what you're talking about when you say, "Alice has an excellent memory." The second form referred to mnemonic techniques to enhance memory. Its name, "artificial memory," not only connoted an alternative to natural memory but also carried the meaning of "artful," an activity that requires imagination and creativity, the essential components of the memory arts. We have seen examples in the Memory Lab.

Cicero excelled at both forms of memory. But what about the rest of us who wish to improve our memory? His distinction identifies two possible paths we can take. We might seek to improve our natural memory by strengthening the basic hardware underlying working memory and other memory systems. Or we could accept the natural memory we have and focus instead on mnemonic strategies for demanding situations. This chapter examines both paths.

The First Path: Improving Natural Memory

One intuitively appealing way to strengthen natural memory is to do the same thing we do to build strength in a muscle—exercise. The idea has a checkered history. Some early Romans believed that rote memorization aided the memory system as a whole. Quintilian, a respected educator and orator of the first century A.D., was a proponent of this view:

> If I am asked what is the one great art of memory, the answer is "practice and effort." The most important thing is to learn a lot by heart and think a lot out without writing, if possible every day. No other faculty is so much developed by practice or impaired by neglect. And so not only should children learn as much as possible by heart, but students of any age should be willing to swallow the initially wearisome business of repeating over and over again what they have written or read [to retain it verbatim in memory].

Quintilian saw a benefit from "practice and effort" not only for rote learning but for memory of all sorts. As in training a muscle, the strength that is developed could be used for any purpose. This belief persisted well into the nineteenth century. William James was the first to put the idea to the test by carrying out an experiment on himself in the 1880s. First, he memorized 158 lines of a French poem by studying it in sessions spread over eight days. The total time required for mastery worked out to fifty seconds per line. Next he undertook to train his memory by learning verbatim the first part of the seventeenth-century English epic poem *Paradise Lost*. This was no small feat—it took him thirty-eight days, working twenty minutes a day, to commit the eight hundred lines to memory. Then he returned to the French poem to see if he could learn the next 150 lines more quickly as a result of his *Paradise Lost* training sessions. It turns out he could not. In fact, the total time was longer, working out to fifty-seven seconds per line. James's prodigious effort failed to support the theory that rote memorization could improve memory in general.

Early twentieth-century psychologists followed up with more sophisticated research designs. Interestingly, they found that gains occurred only when the material used to test memory was similar to the material used for memorization practice. When the test and training material were different, training didn't help. This was what had happened to William James. The fluid, rhyming French poem he used to test his memory was nothing like the stilted, unrhymed English poem of his training sessions. Edward Thorndike, a leader in the early research, concluded that students who practice memorizing Shakespearean sonnets can expect to get better at learning sonnets, but their gains in learning names, dates, numbers, or

Bible verses will be minimal. The limits of memorization training were clear. It allowed people to learn strategies applicable to specific materials, but it had no effect on overall memory.

This view of basic memory was dominant for most of the twentieth century. What the ancients called "natural memory" and what I refer to as core memory functions seemed to be fixed for a given individual. No compelling evidence was unearthed that the core processes themselves could be strengthened. For most of the last 100 years, memory training has been about mastering memory strategies, not about improving core memory.

Then, as the twentieth century drew to a close, three new approaches burst on the scene and reopened an issue that had seemed long settled.

Enter the Computer

The proliferation of personal computers and video games offered possibilities for a new type of mental training. Scientists asked, what would happen if a game were specifically created to improve a useful cognitive ability like working memory? If a program of exercises could indeed produce improvement in working memory, an improvement that strengthened its core processes, the benefits could be substantial because the working memory system is associated with other important cognitive abilities, from reading comprehension to fluid intelligence and reasoning.

An influential test of this approach was published by Swedish researcher Torkel Klingberg and his associates in 2005 in the form of a memory training game developed for children with attention-deficit/hyperactivity disorder (ADHD). Since it was known that working memory deficits play a major role in ADHD, a successful technique for improving working memory could have real educational benefits, not only for this population but also for children with reading disabilities, mathematics handicaps, and language impairments, all of whom show working memory problems.

The training consisted of twenty-five sessions. Each lasted about forty minutes and involved ninety memory exercises based on visual figures, numbers, or letters. For example, a visual memory training exercise began when a four-by-four grid appeared on the screen. Next, one of the sixteen locations turned red for about one second. The red square then moved to a new location for another second and so on for several locations. Then the student was shown a blank grid and asked to click on the spots in the same order or—sometimes—in reverse order.

Klingberg and his associates alternated exercises that emphasized visual memory with others that tested verbal memory for numbers or letters. In every case, the child was required to pay careful attention to memory material and work to retain it. Feedback with reward points and other encouragements gave the test a gamelike feel. A key part of the training was the way Klingberg's computer program altered the game to keep it challenging but not impossible—as the child improved, memory demands went up. A second group of children with ADHD served as a comparison group. They played the same game except that it remained fixed at the easiest level rather than increasing in difficulty as in the first group.

At the end of the training, the children's working memory was tested using tasks different from the ones they had been practicing. The researchers found reliable improvements in the children who played the demanding game but not in the ones assigned to the easy game. Other tests measuring attention and fluid intelligence showed a similar pattern of improvements. Parents (but not teachers) of the children reported fewer ADHD symptoms. Follow-up tests six months later found that the gains were still reliably present.

The Klingberg study showcases the potential power of computer training to target a key cognitive ability—working memory. By providing intensive training that pushed memory demands to the limit, the researchers appeared to have succeeded in improving core memory functions, thus breathing new life into Quintilian's basic assumption. It was a surprising, exciting finding, one suggesting core mental operations could be strengthened if an exercise program targeted them properly.

However, over the years, few similar studies have been as successful. In recent reviews of dozens of computer-training investigations, the results were all over the map. While trainees almost always improved on the working memory tasks they practiced, the training didn't transfer consistently to other working memory situations. Additional problems turned up in follow-up tests, where most studies found the gains short-lived. And when researchers looked at transfer to general cognitive abilities like attention and reasoning, success was rare. The mood in the research community shifted from enthusiasm to a more cautious wait-and-see attitude—and in some cases, outright skepticism.

It's still too early to deliver a verdict on the potential for computer training. Research findings are often messy in a new area of investigation as scientists struggle to get a handle on it. There is no consensus yet about how to do the training, how much is required, or how to measure its effects. It will take time to fine-tune these factors. The potential benefits are great for anyone with deficiencies in working memory—academically underperforming children, older adults, and people who have suffered brain injury. But the proof must be in the pudding, and we will have to wait to learn whether computer training can live up to its promise.

Meanwhile, in a parallel universe, commercial firms began offering training programs to a public that embraced them avidly. In 2009 the market for brain-fitness software was estimated at $265 million and has been projected to reach $1 billion by 2015. The first blockbuster offering was Nintendo's *Brain Age,* followed by a slew of others from such firms as Mindsparke, LearningRx, Posit Science, Lumosity, Jungle Memory, and Cogmed. They are truly a mixed bag. Some were designed by credentialed professionals; others are the work of untrained enthusiasts. Some are stand-alone computer programs; others require a trainer. Some have been used in research studies; others haven't. Some cost little; others cost thousands.

This is a sprawling, competitive, enthusiastic marketplace in which promoters are more than willing to guarantee their customers mental improvements from using their wares. The sellers of Jungle Memory spare no words in asserting that "Jungle Memory is designed to target working memory skills critical for academic success. Jungle Memory can improve reading, writing, and logical processing. It also trains students to pay attention and process information and challenging concepts more quickly." Mindsparke's pitch goes even further: "The focused brain exercise in *Brain Fitness Pro* and *Brain Fitness Pro SE* improves memory, restores brain health, and can reduce the risk of developing Alzheimer's symptoms and dementia. You'll have a better memory in less than three weeks and the benefits of the memory training will last indefinitely."

These are bold claims without independent support. I suspect that for many of the products the truth is much closer to the findings of a massive study carried out by the popular BBC television show "Bang Goes the Theory." More than 10,000 viewers volunteered to be randomly assigned to one of three mental exercise regimens. Two of them were modeled after popular brain-training programs—one focused on reasoning and problem solving, while the other required attention, memory, and fast responding. The third was a control group of people who searched the Internet for answers to trivia questions like "What year did Henry VIII die?" The participants were given tests in memory and reasoning before the training began and then again after the training ended six weeks later. The results, published in the prestigious British journal *Nature*, would not have surprised early psychologists who studied memory training. Participants improved significantly on the skills they practiced, but none of the groups showed meaningful improvements on broader measures of memory and reasoning. Calling a computer program "brain training" doesn't make it so. As Quintilian might have put it, *caveat emptor*, let the buyer beware.

The Buddhist Way: Mindfulness Meditation and Core Memory

In the 1990s, a different approach to mental training emerged when clinical psychologists began to incorporate an ancient Buddhist meditative practice, mindfulness training, into therapies for stress and mood problems.

Mindfulness meditation strives for complete mastery over attention. It has been described as "the awareness that emerges through paying attention on purpose, in the present moment, and nonjudgmentally to the unfolding of experience moment by moment." The idea is to completely experience each ongoing second as it happens and to sustain that awareness over time. As one expert meditator put it, mindfulness is simple but not easy. Attention drifts away from the present to other thoughts and concerns, and once this happens, moments begin to slip past unnoticed. The meditator learns to detect drifts, accept them in a nonjudgmental way, and then gently return attention to the present. It is a demanding top-down process.

Secular versions of mindfulness meditation without mystical overtones became commonplace in North America in the 1970s. About that time, Jon Kabat-Zinn, a professor of medicine at the University of Massachusetts, developed a widely adopted eight-week mindfulness training program for patients suffering from stress related to their medical conditions. The training involved three activities: a sitting meditation with a focus on breathing, a body scan meditation with attention directed around the person, and yoga exercises based on stretching. During meditation, the patients were instructed to remain alert, in the moment, and in control of their attention, all in a gentle and nonjudgmental way. Research showed that they were helped by the training. This success led psychotherapists to incorporate mindfulness training into treatments for depression and other disorders with promising successes. The training has also benefited healthy people without psychological problems who show improved interpersonal relationships and reduced negative emotions.

As mindfulness training became better known to psychologists, cognitive researchers wondered about its effects on core mental processes. When meditators pay close attention to the breathing process, they call on high-level mental operations based on top-down goals and executive control, processes essential to working memory, voluntary attention, and reasoning. Could mindfulness meditation lead to improvements in core mental operations? Researchers have been trying to answer this question, and so far the results are positive. For example, Christian Jensen and his collaborators at the University of Copenhagen taught a group of students mindfulness meditation using the Kabat-Zinn approach and compared its effects to other groups who received either relaxation training or no treatment at all. Before and after the training, all groups took a series of laboratory tests to assess attention, working memory, and perceptual sensitivity. Only the mindfulness group showed a reliable improvement in attention and working memory. They also were able to read rapidly presented letters at shorter exposure speeds, suggesting a speed-up in perception.

Other studies have reported similar benefits, especially for attention. Overall, there is convincing support for the idea that meditators become better able to attend to a task despite distractions and can keep their attention focused for longer periods. These gains not only show up in better test scores, but they also appear as neurological changes in brain areas associated with attention, especially those involved in top-down control and resisting distraction, areas that increase in size and interconnections as a result of meditation.

Memory also seems to profit from mindfulness training. The available studies are generally in agreement with the Jensen finding that working memory is strengthened by the training. In fact, it would be a surprise if this were not the case given working memory's close connection to attention. There also appear to be gains in long-term memory. The researcher Alexandre Heeren and his collaborators looked at the effects of mindfulness training on the ability to remember old personal memories. In one test, they asked people to recall specific events from their lives associated with different cue words like "lucky" or "guilty." The memories of people who had learned to meditate were more specific and detailed after their training. This finding suggests that they were better able to zero in on their memories so they could report them in greater depth.

The bottom line? Mindfulness training looks promising as a way to improve core mental functions, including memory. But it is still too soon to know if the research findings available now will hold up under more scrutiny. Moreover, whether these laboratory gains will translate into real world benefits is an open question.

Body and Mind: Physical Exercise and Core Memory

Everyone knows exercise is good for your body, and recent studies have found that it's also good for mental processes. The evidence is especially convincing from studies of the elderly, which show that exercise is associated with lower rates of mental decline. In one large project, randomly selected Canadians over the age of sixty-five were recruited for a multi-year study. First, researchers assessed their cognitive functioning and their level of physical exercise. Five years later 4,615 of the respondents who had initially tested in the cognitive normal range were located and tested again to look for mental decline as indicated by deficits in memory, thinking, and judgment. Mental decline was as much as twice as likely in those who were inactive.

The Canadian study raised the question of whether sedentary seniors could improve their cognitive functioning by adopting a program of regular exercise. It appears so. Arthur Kramer and his associates divided 124 sedentary seniors between the ages of sixty and seventy-five into two groups. One exercised by walking for forty minutes three times a week for six months, a regimen designed to strengthen aerobic fitness. The other group spent the same amount of time in stretching and toning exercises. When the seniors were assessed at the end, the walking group showed improvements on tests of attention and memory.

These results have been confirmed by other studies. Taken collectively, there is strong support for the conclusion that exercise can improve attention, memory, and processing speed in formerly sedentary older adults. But not just any form of exercise will confer these gains. Successful programs have used either aerobic exercise or strength training, or both. The standout choice for aerobic exercise has been brisk walking for thirty to sixty minutes several times a week. Strength training typically has used free weights or gym equipment. There is some evidence that the combination of aerobic activity and strength training is especially beneficial. What doesn't seem to work is exercise with low energy and slow movements, like stretching.

What about exercise benefits for other age groups? The case is strongest for preadolescent children who show cognitive advantages when they are fit. Those who have high aerobic fitness, as determined by endurance and strength testing, show better academic achievement and better test performance in areas such as attention, planning, and resisting distraction—the high-level processes needed to handle demanding tasks. Neurological studies show that fit children have more brain volume and increased brain activity in structures important for information processing, including memory. A few studies have investigated the benefits of giving sedentary children regular exercise, and the results suggest small improvements in attention, memory, and top-down control. Cognitive effects of exercise for those between adolescence and late middle age have been studied infrequently and are poorly understood. Nonetheless, there are signs of a positive relationship. One study showed that twelve weeks of aerobic exercise improved memory for lengthy word lists in formerly sedentary adults between the ages of twenty-one and forty-five. Brain scans revealed that areas important for long-term memory had been strengthened during the training.

How Much Exercise?

If you decide to exercise regularly to improve your cognitive fitness, what exercises should you do and how long should you do them? There is no precise answer yet, but a reasonable approach is to follow government guidelines. For healthy adults, the recommendation is 150 minutes per week of moderate aerobic exercise equivalent to brisk walking. This is in the ballpark of the various exercise regimens used in research studies, and it works out to an average of about twenty minutes a day—although the 150 minutes can be distributed in any way that is convenient. Strength training is also beneficial, at least for older adults. The same government guidelines recommend strength training for major muscle groups twice a week with activities like weight lifting, calisthenics, or yoga.

Strengthening Natural Memory: Closing Thoughts

What can be said, then, of the prospects for improving your "natural memory"? First, improvements seem possible—this is a departure from the common opinion of twentieth-century researchers, who for the most part treated natural memory as fixed. So, if you want to bump up your core cognitive performance, there's every reason to try one of these approaches. In my own life, I try to maintain a regular program of exercise and meditation for their many possible benefits.

If you undertake one of these strengthening regimens, how much memory improvement can you expect? To answer this question, we first need to look at the tests used to measure the gains. The famous "bell curve" below is an idealized representation of how people score on tests of memory. Most people score in the middle range, with smaller numbers scoring higher or lower. The point marked "50th Percentile" means that fifty percent of test takers have this score or a lower one.

Now, suppose your initial score on a test of working memory was at the fiftieth percentile and you complete one of the better researched programs of computer exercises. Where would you move to on the bell curve? The next curve, shown on the facing page, is based on average gains found in available research studies and shows you could expect your scores to move up to the seventy-fourth percentile, the line marked *a*. This is a notable improvement all right, but then it is based on the kinds of tests you have been practicing on the computer. When different working memory tests are given to determine how well improvements transfer to other situations, the gains drop to the fifty-fifth percentile, shown as point *c*.

What would happen if you are a sedentary senior and undertake a pro-

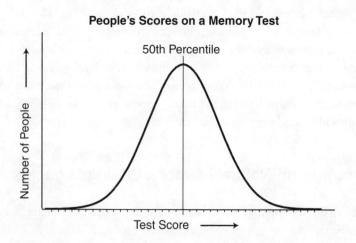

People's Scores on a Memory Test

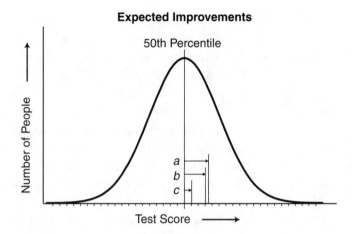

gram of regular exercise? You could expect your working memory score to move from the fiftieth to the seventy-first percentile relative to other sedentary seniors, the point marked b. Note, though, that working memory improvements from exercise are often not seen in people who are younger and more fit. If you decided to practice meditation and stay with it, you could expect an improvement in working memory that would bump you from the fiftieth to the seventy-second percentile, near point b on the bell curve.

You will need to work hard to realize these gains; it may take weeks or months to achieve them. You will likely need periodic refresher workouts to maintain any improvements you attain; just how often and how extensive the refreshers need to be have yet to be determined. Also keep in mind that these are gains on laboratory tests. Improvements in day-to-day memory performance may or may not be obvious. But the potential for improvement is real for those who carry out these regimens. And you may find your efforts in computer games, exercise, or meditation rewarding, regardless of their impact on your memory.

The Second Path: Mnemonic Technique

Now we turn to the other path to memory improvement, the path the ancients called "artificial memory," an approach based on the memory arts. Without question, dramatic gains are possible for those who become skilled in their use. Recall Joshua Foer, who learned to memorize a deck of cards in less than two minutes, or Harry Lorayne, who learned the names of everyone in large audiences. Their specialized techniques, based on various Dragon Principles, allowed them to repackage and organize memory material so that they could retain it better. And you don't have to be a professional mnemonist to use such memory aids. When you're introduced to "Mr. Collins," you might imagine a friendly *collie* jumping on him, thus immediately transforming a random pairing between a name and a person into an active, meaningful association and a memory you can more easily retain. The long and distinguished history of mnemonic techniques is testimony to their practicality. Even Quintilian, with his enthusiasm for rote memorization, endorsed the memory arts and taught them to his students, as did other teachers before and after him.

But the memory arts are neither a silver bullet nor a free lunch. They must be tailored to each situation and applied deliberately. This means that the techniques useful for remembering names will be of little help in remembering numbers—they require different strategies. And each technique has its own learning curve that must be followed before proficiency is achieved. This requires discipline, focus, and effort because the memory arts depend on high-level cognitive operations—attention, top-down control, and mental manipulations in working memory. Consider how you would create the memory image for remembering Mr. Collins's name. You begin with a conscious decision to find the mnemonic. Next, you would have to search your memory for a concrete word that sounds similar to his name. Once you decide on "collie," you must generate an image of the dog jumping on Mr. Collins.

For the practitioner of the memory arts, though, the required effort has an upside. In addition to the obvious benefit of creating stronger memories, the memory arts challenge you to use your wits, to think on your feet, and to improve your ability to use your own mental resources. Indeed, you may find that the most significant rewards won't come from the names you remember or the facts you master. The richer rewards may be a sense of accomplishment and confidence in your mental capabilities. We live in a time of devices that make our life easier but often dramatically lower intellectual demands. Google not only searches out facts for me; it even helps spell the search terms I use. The memory arts are a movement in the opposite direction. They are about intellectual self-reliance; they offer a sense of control over your environment that can be both stimulating and satisfying.

The remainder of the book examines memory strategies for specific situations. You will discover what science has revealed about making information and events memorable, about preserving them over time, and about recalling them when you need them. You will understand why some situations give you trouble and how you can draw on your memory system's strengths to deal with them. You will see how to apply the Dragon Principles and other memory insights in diverse settings.

In the Memory Lab:
Creating Effective Visual Associations

Visual mnemonics rely on an association between a visual cue and the target memory it is intended to retrieve. This Memory Lab is a case study that shows a common error in selecting visual cues. Take a look at the visual mnemonic below, which was devised to help retain the idea that there are two paths for improving memory.

You can see what the creator of the mnemonic had in mind. The brain image was intended to cue ways to improve natural memory by strengthening core processes, and the palette was intended to cue the memory arts. The mnemonist also made one path broad and the other narrow to cue the idea that the memory arts are situation-specific while improvements to natural memory are global.

So what is the error? The weakness is that the brain image provides no help whatsoever in recalling the three different ways to strengthen natural memory. Why did the mnemonist choose the brain

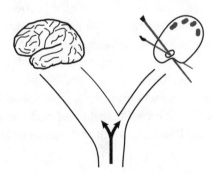

A proposed mnemonic to cue the two paths to memory improvement.

image as a cue? If we retrace his thought process, we will gain an important insight about creating mnemonics.

The mnemonist likely began searching for a cue that would help recall the three ways to improve core memory functions by thinking of associations to the different ways. As he thought about it, he zeroed in on brain changes as the common associate of all three. That is:

computer training → brain strengthening
meditation → brain strengthening
exercise → brain strengthening

At the time the mnemonist created the mnemonic, the brain seemed a logical associate of the three methods. The problem is that when he uses the mnemonic, the association must work in the opposite direction if he is to recall all three: That is, he will recall the mnemonic and think: brain → ?? This is where the mnemonic comes up short.

His mistake is an easy error to make and a common source of ineffective mnemonics: a cue that seemed useful and reasonable when the mnemonic was created turns out to be weak when the mnemonic is used, because the direction of association has been reversed.

At the time of mnemonic creation:
    memory material → think of memory cue
At the time of mnemonic use:
    memory cue → think of memory material

What this means for you as a mnemonist is that you need to be sensitive to the direction of association between a memory cue and the memory material—the association has to work when you use the mnemonic, not when you create it.

What could the mnemonist have done instead? The image on the facing page is an alternative. The cue for improving natural memory now suggests a computer game showing a Buddha meditating with athletic shoes attached to the game console for exercising. It is a mnemonic that can allow rapid recall of the three interventions.

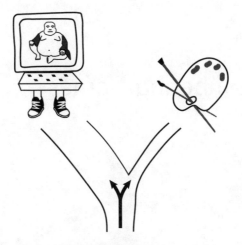

An improved mnemonic with more specific cues.

7

Remembering Names

I was at a party, and I spotted a former coworker I hadn't seen for a while. I went over, along with my date, and we started to talk. He introduced his wife and I introduced my date. It was only a little later that I turned to his wife to ask about her work, and I realized I had completely forgotten her name. It was simply gone. I was embarrassed, but I faked it, and I don't think she knew. Later I heard her introduced to someone else, and then I had it.

A student in one of my classes told me this story, which describes a predicament familiar to most of us. In fact, surveys find that forgetting names is the most common memory complaint, and it doesn't matter whether you're asking college students or older adults, although laments grow louder as we age.

There are good reasons that names cause problems. Often we first hear a name at a busy social event where there are lots of distractions. And some names are unfamiliar, which can make them slippery. But there is also another factor at work. It turns out that there is something about names that makes them hard to remember even when the name is easy and even when we give it full attention. Names are difficult just because they are names.

Consider the two people shown as cartoons on the facing page: Mr. Farmer, the attorney, and Mr. Roberts, the farmer. Now suppose you meet these two at a gathering and hear their names and their occupations. Are you more likely to forget "farmer" when you hear it as a name or as an occupation?

Researcher Lori James studied memory for words like "farmer" that

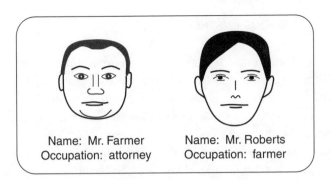

can be either a person's name or a person's occupation. She found that when a word is used as a name, it is instantly more difficult to remember. She gave her research participants the job of learning the name and occupation of individuals depicted in pictures. She used words like "farmer," "baker," "weaver," and "cook" so she could give some participants the word as a name and others the same word as an occupation, similar to the cartoons. She included both college students and senior citizens in the study to examine age effects. Later, people were shown the pictures and asked to give the name and occupation of each person. The results were clear cut, as the bar graph below shows: when a word was presented as an occupation, it was well remembered, but when it was presented as a name, it was not. As expected, the older adults had more difficulty than the younger group with names. Neither group had trouble remembering occupations.

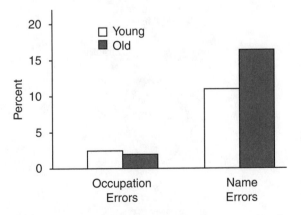

Memory for names and memory for occupations are quite different.

What Is It about Names?

Why is a word that's easy to remember as an occupation so much harder to remember as a name? The answer to this question provides an insight into the memory system and suggests workable strategies for learning names. It all comes down to the associations available when you retrieve the word as shown in the drawing below. When I tell you that Mr. Roberts is a farmer, you immediately know quite a bit about him—he can drive a tractor, grow crops, and work a field. Later, if you want to recall his occupation and it doesn't immediately come to mind, you will probably remember some of the other associations, that he drives a tractor, for example, and it will cue the fact that he is a farmer.

But when you try to recall his name, there is only one path. There are no additional associations—a name is just an arbitrary designator for a person and carries no extra meaning. It doesn't matter whether it's "Roberts" or "Cook." If the single link connecting the name to the person is weak, you'll have trouble remembering the name. There is no Plan B.

So how can you improve your memory for names? The drawing below shows the three requirements to make that happen. You have to remember the face, the name, and the connection among them. If any one of these memories is weak, you could be reduced to a blank look when it comes time to recall the name. We will see effective strategies that help ensure that doesn't happen, and we begin with an especially important step.

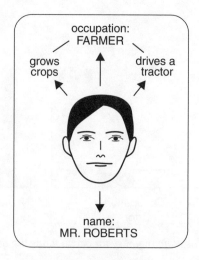

Remembering the Person

Remembering a name will be pointless unless it is somehow connected to the person. Usually this means associating the name with the person's face, the body part most associated with our identity. If you are one of those people who seldom forgets a face, even after a brief encounter, count yourself lucky. For the rest of us, there are ways to improve our face memory. This is the essential first step in boosting the ability to remember names.

Faces are not ordinary visual objects, like a shoe, or even like another part of the body like an arm or a leg. Faces are the first thing babies focus on, and throughout life faces give us crucial information to help us identify people, size them up, infer their moods, and guess their intentions. It is because the face is so important that some researchers believe specialized neural circuitry has evolved for analyzing and remembering it, circuitry that makes use of two different aspects of the face for identification. We may use specific individual features—a big nose or attractive eyes. Or we may rely on our impression of all the features taken together. When you first meet a person, specific facial features are often the most important factor for recognizing that person again. That is why you may fail to identify a woman you met recently if she has a new hairstyle or has gone from blond to brunette. But if you interact with her over and over, you become familiar with the overall layout of her face and perceive it holistically. Now if she changes her hair, you take it in stride—you may be surprised, but you won't be confused about who she is.

Because holistic perception of the face can be weak when you meet a new person, it is a good strategy to seek out a specific feature—the strong jaw line or the close-set eyes—to connect the person with the name. As the face becomes more familiar, the name will eventually become associated with its holistic properties, but that will take care of itself in due time. The advice of professional mnemonists is right in line with this approach—zero in on a distinguishing facial feature to associate with the name. According to memory masters Harry Lorayne and Jerry Lucas,

> What you select could be anything: hair or hairline, forehead (narrow, wide, or high); eyebrows (straight, arched, bushy); eyes (narrow, wide-spaced, close-set); nose (large, small, pug, ski); nostrils (flaring, pinched); high cheekbones; cheeks (full or sunken); lips (straight, arched, full, thin); chin (cleft, receding, jutting); lines, pimples, warts, dimples—anything.

To make this work, you have to look closely at the face, and that is not something all of us do routinely. If you are casual about focusing on facial details, you will need to make an extra effort here. Lorayne and Lucas suggest that you give special weight to your first impressions as you *really look* at the face. The bushy eyebrows you notice when you first meet Spencer will likely catch your attention again when you see him next time. This is just what you want to connect Spencer to his name.

What If You Can't Find a Distinctive Feature?

When no feature pops out at the time of the introduction, it is likely no feature will pop out the next time you see the person. So instead of going for a feature, try for a holistic, overall impression of the face and use that to associate with the name. Focus on the center of the face just below the eyes and give full attention to the way the face is configured, not in terms of the specifics but overall. The deep processing you do as you study the face will also help you remember it.

Other stable personal qualities can be used to connect the person to the name—say, weight or height or a particular personality style. A nervous manner, a fat belly, hairy arms, scarlet nails can all be memory cues if you pay attention to them. You can even use clothing or jewelry, especially at one-shot events where you are unlikely to interact with the person again. Big loop earrings or a cobalt blue shirt can be all you need to link the individual and the name for the event.

Problems Remembering Faces?

People differ significantly in their ability to recognize faces. One study found a sevenfold difference among college students in face–memory problems, difficulties such as mistaking one person for another or failing to recognize someone they knew well.

You can improve your skill at remembering faces—and thus names—by making a deliberate effort to attend to them and identify distinguishing features. Practice doing this in a setting where there is a steady stream of people—a shopping mall or a busy sidewalk. As a person passes, take a careful look at the face and select a distinguishing feature or, if none jumps out at you, try for a holistic impression. After you pass several people—start with two or three—recall the faces and the memory cues you picked.

You will find the task gets easier with practice. As memory expert Kenneth Higbee observed, "Actually, there are many distinguishing features in a face, but you have to train yourself to look for them. Once you do, you will see much more in a face."

Creating a Strong Name–Person Connection: The Basics

Now we are ready to put it all together and take up the full process of connecting a person to a name. I recommend that you always begin with a retention intention—a personal commitment to retain the name and a plan for doing it. Your commitment to get the name is crucial. Make it something you want to happen by giving yourself a reason—maybe it's to make a good impression, or maybe you see learning the name as a challenge, an opportunity to exercise your mental powers. It can also help to deliberately make yourself interested in the person you are about to meet. Who *is* this guy? What's his story? You won't learn all that in the introduction, of course, but you can size him up and learn his name. Tactics like these increase focus and motivation.

While you are at it, decide just what part of the name you want to remember. In most social situations, if I say, "My name is Bob Madigan," "Bob" is all you need to retain. On the other hand, if you are meeting me as your new professor, "Madigan" is the important part. In either case, you only need to remember part of what you hear, and this makes the task easier.

Now for specific strategies. The first approach is one that ensures good encoding and a strong connection between face and name. It is easy to apply and gives real benefit. If you take only one idea from this chapter, make it this one. This name-learning process has four steps: Find a Feature, Listen, Say, and Practice. I suggest you remember it as an acrostic: Friendly Llamas Seek People. Its helper image is shown on the next page.

Find a Feature

Decide as quickly as you can on the feature you will use to connect the person with the name so you can lower your cognitive load during the actual introduction. Often you can spot people you are likely to be introduced to

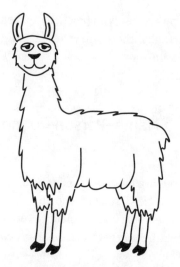

A helper image for the acrostic Friendly Llamas Seek People.

well before you meet them. This is a good time to look them over and find something about them to connect with their names when the time comes. Will it be a specific facial feature? Some other feature? A holistic impression?

Listen

A lapse in attention during an introduction spells real trouble, and it can easily happen in busy settings. You need firm top-down control of attention to make sure the name is well registered in your memory. Seniors appear to be especially vulnerable to problems here because they are more susceptible to distractions that derail attention. If you didn't hear the name well, ask the person to repeat it. Some people find this awkward because it interrupts the flow of the introduction, but it's necessary if you want to learn the name. I find people don't mind at all if I ask them to say their name again—it shows my interest in meeting them.

Say

Plan to repeat the name—"Nice to meet you, Emma." Getting in the habit of doing this is valuable because it involves retrieval practice, one of the most powerful ways to strengthen memory. And by listening to yourself as you say "Emma," you hear the name again.

Practice

This is a key to success. It strengthens memory for the name and the selected feature while forging a connection between them. The first retrieval practice takes place when you repeat the name, but usually this is not enough. Get additional practice by looking at the person, noticing the feature you chose, and recalling the name. Take advantage of opportunities to use the new name in conversation. This can be overdone, of course, but you don't have to actually say the name out loud; you can do it mentally, as in "Good point (Roger)." Each time you practice the name and note the chosen feature, you strengthen their association.

Mnemonist Scott Hagwood recommends three rehearsals within five minutes of learning the name, and research is consistent with his advice. Psychologist Peter Morris and his colleagues asked people to learn new names both in the laboratory and at a real party by practicing them three times. Under laboratory conditions, three retrieval practices boosted name retention by two hundred percent. In the real world, with its many distractions, the gain dropped to fifty percent, still a major improvement.

When you need to retain the name–face association longer than the event, more practice is in order. How extensive it should be depends on how long it will be before you meet the person again. If it will be relatively soon—a few days, perhaps—then one more retrieval practice late in the day of the introduction may well be enough. The drill is to think back to the person, visualize the feature, and recall the name. But if the retention interval will be longer, use the Rule of Five discussed in Chapter 4 as a guide to decide how you will keep the memory strong.

More Powerful Name–Face Associations

When Harry Lorayne amazed audiences by learning all their names, he used advanced techniques. He couldn't rely on retrieval practice because there was no time for it. Instead, he retained the names by creating vivid visual imagery that connected names to appearance, imagery powerful enough to remember the names without rehearsal.

There is no question about the efficacy of this approach when it's used by a skilled mnemonist. In my experience, it is the best way to capture a new name because the vivid associations require less maintenance to keep them strong. It not only helps you remember the name, but it can also encode a connection between the name and the chosen feature. The downside is that the imagery associations require more effort and cognitive resources than the Friendly Llama strategy, sometimes more than you can manage. Think of these advanced methods as add-ons to the Friendly Llama steps, optional enhancements that will help if you can pull them off.

The "Shadow Technique" for First Names

Often we know someone who has the same first name as the person being introduced. Take "Spencer" for example. I know a Spencer, and I can use this knowledge to learn the name of a new Spencer I have just met by visualizing the Spencer I know slapping the back of the new Spencer. With a little practice, you can do this quickly, using acquaintances, celebrities, or politicians as shadows.

The most powerful associations will be those in which the shadow image interacts with the target person's distinctive feature, such as visualizing old Spencer pulling on new Spencer's bushy eyebrows. An image like this not only helps you remember Spencer's name; it connects it to his distinguishing feature, an ideal memory cue. But sometimes I find this technique too complicated, and I settle for creating a good image of the shadow slapping the person on the back, or locking arms with the person, or even just looking over the new person's shoulder. This helps me remember the name, and then I rely on retrieval practice to strengthen the association with the person's distinguishing feature.

Techniques for Last Names

You can sometimes use the shadow technique with last names. If you meet Mr. Sullivan and you remember your high school pal Rick Sullivan, by all means take advantage of it and create the shadow. Another lucky break is when the last name can be interpreted as a meaningful word—Ms. Farmer, Mr. Gardner, or Ms. Castle. Here the strategy is to fashion an image around the word that connects the person with the meaning in the name. You might imagine Ms. Farmer in overalls or holding a pitchfork. In the same way, you could imagine Mr. Hoover operating a vacuum cleaner and Ms. Brown wearing a big floppy brown hat. Or you may notice that Ms. Clay has very curly hair, and so you could picture her at a potter's wheel with bits of clay flying into her hair. This last example ties together her distinguishing feature and an image suggesting her name. It is a home run as a name-feature memory image.

Unfortunately, last names usually do not directly translate into an image, and then the "substitute word" technique becomes the only option. We saw this in Chapter 1 where I converted "episodic" and "semantic" into the memory cue "exotic salmon." This strategy is especially useful for names. So, when you meet Mr. Roberts, look for a concrete word that sounds enough like his name to be a useful memory cue. Perhaps you come up with "robber" as shown in the drawing below. You might imagine him carrying a bag of burglary tools. If you create a good image to bring "robber" to mind, you will have an associative link to his name that will greatly improve your chances of remembering it.

Here are other examples. I notice Mr. Burrill is tall and athletic; I imagine him carrying a surprised *burro*. I picture Ms. Gurke *gargling*, Mr. Luzano surrounded by *loose ammo*, Ms. Kopischke as a cop (*"cop is me"*), Mr. Boydston as a fat kid (*"boy ton"*), Ms. Arnell with an *arm bell*, and Mr. Tillman *tilling* his garden. Professor Madigan could be pictured as getting *mad again*. These images provide the most help when they include an inter-

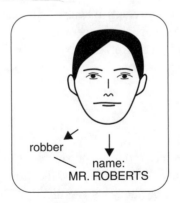

How a substitute word for a name adds an associative link that improves name memory.

action with the person's distinctive feature, as was the case with Mr. Burrill.

Developing a knack for turning a name into an image takes practice. Try to go into name–image mode every time you meet a new person. Think of it as a game—the way the punster delights in finding hidden meanings in words or the rapper enjoys generating rhymes. While it's unlikely that you will be able to convert every name to an image, you can certainly improve your ability. And as this happens, you will see your memory for names take a quantum jump.

Laboratory studies show that both college students and senior citizens improved name–face memory using this strategy. This technique has also seen enduring popularity in practical memory training programs, most notably those offered by Harry Lorayne, who has taught it to generations of corporate executives, celebrities, military officers, and other audiences, as well as describing it in memory improvement books. Other experienced memory trainers teach similar methods.

Be warned, though: mastering the imagery method takes effort. It's especially challenging in fast-moving social situations where it can be hard to marshal the mental resources to find the concrete words and create the imagery. In two studies in which students had learned the approach in the laboratory and then tried to use it in real life, the method did not help them. But the students were novices—they had just been taught the techniques—and with more practice they would surely have improved. The lesson from this research is that mastery of this powerful method takes time. My advice is to attempt to form a name–feature image when you carry out the basic Friendly Llama strategy. When you can readily convert the name to an image, by all means use the image, but if one is not forthcoming, continue with the default plan and rely on retrieval practice to retain the name, the feature, and their association.

Many Names

You walk into a conference room at a prospective client's office. Eight men and women are seated around a table—and the introductions begin. "John, I'd like you to meet Harry, and this is Sally. . . . " Each person nods or reaches across to shake your hand. When it comes to remembering names, no setting is more daunting. The situation moves too fast for retrieval practice, and you can just feel the names slipping away. But there are steps you can take to cope with group introductions, whether at a meeting or a party or other social event where you meet many people.

Here is the primary rule: Don't give up. When you're having trouble keeping all the names straight, it's easy to just stop trying. But if you can hang in there and apply the Friendly Llama strategy as well as you can, you will likely retain some of the names long enough to get through the introductions when retrieval practice is possible. Often you can pick up the ones you forgot if you pay attention during the event.

There are also specific strategies that can be helpful. For example, you might be able to squeeze in a little rehearsal practice if you work at it. As each new person is introduced, follow the Friendly Llama strategy, and then before you are introduced to the next person, glance at the one you met before the current person and say the name to yourself. As soon as the introductions are complete, look for more opportunities to practice.

Another technique was suggested by Don Gabor, a business coach and motivational speaker. He calls it the "letter chain," and it goes like this. As each person is introduced, build an acronym from the first letters of the names. If you first meet Cameron and then Haley, remember C–H. Next you're introduced to Alex, and the acronym becomes C–H–A. As soon as you can, look at the people and run through the names to practice them. The letter chain is helpful up to three or four names before it starts getting too cumbersome.

The Name Game

There is an ingenious technique that allows an entire group to learn everyone's name. Called the "name game," it works best in settings where there is someone in charge who can direct it. The game begins when the first person says his or her name. The next group member says the first person's name before giving his or her own name. The "game" continues like this around the room, each person saying all the preceding names before a self-introduction. The other group members are encouraged to play along silently, and if someone gets stuck, help comes from the group. When a blackboard is available, each person writes his or her name on the board before saying it and then erases the board.

In addition to boosting memory, the name game is fun. It can break the ice and allow people to make connections with each other. Researchers

Peter Morris and Catherine Fritz have found that people remember three times as many names using the game as they do with standard introductions, a success rate that comes from the retrieval practice it provides. It seems to work best in groups up to about a dozen, although Morris and Fritz have used it with as many as twenty-five.

A Final Thought

A good memory for names has many benefits. In occupations where customer service or networking is important, the person who remembers the names of contacts has a real advantage over those who don't. As Dale Carnegie observed back in 1936, "Remember that a man's name is to him the sweetest and most important sound in the English language." Knowing someone's name establishes a link with the person that can pay dividends in just about any social situation because it establishes a personal connection. I get a striking reminder of this in my role as college instructor. At the beginning of a new term, I try to learn the students' names in the first few classes, and once that happens there is always a palpable change in my experience at the podium. The class becomes transformed from a sea of faces to a group of individuals, because I have a connection to each person. Surprisingly, this happens even though I don't know a specific thing about the students other than their names. You may find, as I have, that there is a special gratification in applying memory techniques to names and faces.

In the next chapter, we examine another memory setting that has both practical benefits and personal satisfaction. We look at ways to remember to carry out a future action, like picking up the dry cleaning on the way home. We will see why these situations can be challenging and how memory strategies can improve the chances that we won't arrive home empty-handed.

In the Memory Lab: Learning from Forgetting

The habit of learning people's names not only has social rewards but is an excellent way to hone memory skills in general as you exercise key mnemonic operations such as attention, top-down control, imagery, creativity, fast thinking, and rehearsal. Because it is challenging, you won't always be successful. In this installment of the Memory

Lab, we look at a fact of life for the practitioner of the memory arts: occasional memory failures. My message here is that these failures can sharpen your memory skills if you approach them in the right way. In fact, I believe failures can contribute as much or more to improving memory skill as successes.

To reap this benefit, you have to view memory failure as a problem with your technique, not a sign of a global memory shortcoming. Say you forgot two of the four names you heard at the beginning of the meeting. It won't help to ask yourself, "What's wrong with my memory?" or to think, "Uh-oh, another senior moment." Thoughts like these make you worry about your basic memory ability, and they do nothing to enhance your memory in the future. In fact, they may have just the opposite effect because they feed negative expectations that can easily become self-fulfilling prophecies.

What should you do instead? First, accept and own the memory failure. Next, conduct a postmortem to figure out what went wrong. Was it inattention? Information overload? Weak imagery? Inadequate rehearsal? Poorly focused memory retrieval? If you can pin the problem down, you may be able to think of a better way to handle a similar situation in the future. I say "may" because not every memory failure is preventable. Sometimes memory demands simply exceed memory skill. But often you may find that you can come up with a better way to handle the situation, and when you can, you have an opportunity to improve your skill. Try not to waste failures.

8

Remembering to Remember

Memory can be about the future as well as the past. You intend to mail that gift after work, or pay the phone bill before Wednesday, or meet with your nephew Justin at three o'clock. Psychologists call this "prospective memory"; it's about remembering to carry out an action. It helps us stay healthy, manage our relationships, and be productive in our work.

Prospective memory is a particularly fallible form of memory. By one estimate, over half of the daily memory problems people experience involve prospective memory. Most of them are inconsequential—forgetting the dry cleaning, leaving the porch light on, even missing a staff meeting or showing up for a lecture without the handouts. Although irritating and embarrassing, these are minor inconveniences. But not all prospective memory errors are benign. Because prospective memory is about actions, there can be serious consequences to forgetting.

One startling case in point had its roots in the well-intentioned effort to improve child safety in cars. Studies showed that children are less at risk for injury in an accident if they are in the back seat, and in the 1990s laws were passed mandating that child safety seats be secured there. But this made it possible for a distracted driver, intending to drop a child off at daycare on the way somewhere else, to forget about the child in the back seat and leave the child in a parked car. In summer months especially, this can be a deadly memory error. Although precise numbers aren't known, experts estimate between fifteen and twenty-five children die each year when their busy parents forget them in a closed car in the heat.

How could such a prospective memory error occur? What kind of parent would succumb to it? *Washington Post* writer Gene Weingarten, who investigated a number of these cases, discovered who does it.

The wealthy do, it turns out. And the poor, and the middle class. Parents of all ages and ethnicities do it. Mothers are just as likely to do it as fathers. It happens to the chronically absent-minded and to the fanatically organized, to the college educated and to the marginally literate. In the last 10 years, it has happened to a dentist. A postal clerk. A social worker. A police officer. An accountant. A soldier. A paralegal. An electrician. A Protestant clergyman. A rabbinical student. A nurse. A construction worker. An assistant principal. It happened to a mental health counselor, a college professor, and a pizza chef. It happened to a pediatrician. It happened to a rocket scientist.

Indeed, these incidents are less about the weaknesses of specific people than about a weakness of memory. After reading Weingarten's full account, which won a Pulitzer Prize, it is hard to escape the conclusion that any of us could blunder into a situation like this where, under the right conditions, our prospective memory could stumble, with catastrophic results.

How Prospective Memory Fails

When the parents left for these fatal drives, the possibility that a horrific event could occur never entered their minds. They implicitly assumed that the thought to drop the child off would occur to them at the proper time just as it always had in the past. But in fact they were dependent on a memory trigger kicking in to cue the dropoff. Although there were a number of ways a cuing trigger could have occurred, none of them worked.

To understand the cuing process, first step back and look at the prime mover behind a prospective memory, the intention to perform the future act—in this case, to drop off the child on the way to work. The intention serves as memory for the action, but this is no ordinary memory, because it involves a goal along with a plan and motivation to carry it out. Sophisticated studies show that an intention, once made, remains active in the background of the cognitive system even when the person is not thinking about it, and that active status appears to be retained until the goal is either accomplished or abandoned. Sigmund Freud captured the idea long ago when he wrote that an intention "slumbers on in the person until time for execution approaches. Then it awakes and impels him to perform the action."

But just what "awakens" the intention? This question is at the crux of much prospective memory research. Mark McDaniel and Gilles Einstein, prominent investigators in the area, proposed that cues to carry out an intention can be detected through either top-down or bottom-up processes. The distinction is whether we make an effort to search for the cues or just wait for them to pop into consciousness.

In a top-down scenario, we deliberately stay alert until the cue occurs, a process called active monitoring. It is the strategy of choice when we anticipate that it will be hard to notice the cue. So if you intend to say hello to an old friend at the annual cocktail reception of the Friends of the Library, you are likely to be on the lookout for her with active monitoring as you participate in the event. We use the same strategy when the planned action is especially important. If you intend to stop for gas on the way home because the tank is down to fumes, you are likely to stay alert for a station. In both cases, the top-down process of active monitoring improves the chances of carrying out the intended task, although it by no means guarantees it. Not only can active monitoring be derailed by a lapse in attention; it can also run into trouble when you do something else while you are staying alert for the cue. At the cocktail party you run into your brother-in-law and get absorbed in a conversation about next year's funding drive as you keep an eye out for your friend. Active monitoring requires the top-down resources of the frontal lobes. If the conversation also needs these resources, something has to give, and the result is performance problems either in finding your friend or in carrying on the discussion, or both. For all its advantages, active monitoring is a demanding, mentally costly way to detect a cue to perform an intended action.

This is why it is unlikely that the parents of the forgotten children were actively looking for the road to the daycare center on the day of the tragic trip. They didn't view the dropoff as anything out of the ordinary; it was just another routine stop on a routine trip. If any of them had thought, even for a second, their child would be harmed if they missed the road, they surely would have actively watched for it and made the stop. But that wasn't their mindset. Instead, they relied on the second way we trigger an intended action—a bottom-up process that automatically responds to a cue and triggers memory for the action, a process called spontaneous retrieval. This is what researchers McDaniel and Einstein believe is our preferred way to deal with prospective situations.

For the parents, spontaneous retrieval was likely at the point where they needed to alter the route and make a turn toward the daycare center. A landmark like this provides the driver with a cue that (1) is pertinent for driving and (2) connects with the prospective intention. Researchers call this a "focal cue" because it is relevant for both the driving task and the intention, a combination that makes spontaneous retrieval especially likely. But "likely" isn't the same as certain, and on these tragic trips it didn't happen.

After missing the turn, the odds of remembering the daycare stop became much lower, although spontaneous retrieval was still possible. Perhaps noticing another daycare center along the road could have retrieved the intention, but this would be a long shot because it is a nonfocal cue, one not relevant to driving. A random thought could have led to spontaneous retrieval, but it didn't happen this time. The last chance to trigger the intention was when the driver parked at the final destination and closed up the car, but the cue the driver needed, the baby in the back seat, was nonfocal, and so the disaster script played out.

This analysis of prospective memory shows that it is anything but a sure bet when we are occupied with other matters and not actively monitoring. Success is completely dependent on encountering a trigger for the "slumbering" intention, a requirement that can be problematic indeed. Overconfidence can also contribute to a failure. We tend to approach these situations with assurance: Of course I will remember to pay that bill today. Of course I will remember to mail the gift. Of course I will remember the three o'clock meeting. But the truth is we don't always remember, and we find ourselves surprised and chagrined when active monitoring fails and spontaneous retrieval doesn't occur.

Thus it is prudent to approach prospective memory situations with a modicum of humility. While usually successful, prospective memory is inherently error prone. Fortunately, there are steps you can take to improve its operation. You can create better external cues for the action. Alternatively, you can make mental preparations to help trigger the intention at the right moment.

Improving Prospective Memory with External Cues

We all use external memory aids for prospective memory. Need to mail a letter tomorrow? Put it next to the car keys. Need to take a pill at breakfast? Put it in the cup you use for coffee. Have an appointment later today? Put a sticky note on your computer screen.

The idea is to find a stimulus that will prompt spontaneous retrieval of the intention and locate it where it becomes a focal cue. Such ploys work. The most powerful external cues are those that are connected directly to the intended action, like the letter placed by the keys or the pill in the cup. But even generic cues can be effective. The classic remedy for prospective memory is a string around the finger. The assumption is that it will periodically catch your attention and remind you of what you planned to do. But the string itself is a generic cue and conveys nothing about just what it is that needs doing.

While actually tying a string on a finger is rare, I have seen people wear a watch upside down, move a ring to the opposite hand, rest a backpack in an unusual position, and devise other creative attention grabbers. These are interesting memory aids because they show we often don't need to be reminded of the specific action as much as we need to be reminded that there is *something* we intend to do. Once we get to that realization, we can search our memory to discover what it is. If the task is at all important, we will likely recall it.

An external cue, either specific or generic, is especially worth considering when the cost of forgetting is high—as in the daycare dropoff—or in a situation where forgetting seems likely, such as taking an important medication. These are times when it's best to acknowledge the frailty of prospective memory and arrange memory aids. To reduce the risk of a forgotten baby, one recommendation is to put needed work papers in the back seat to establish a fail-safe focal cue.

But not all circumstances permit adding an external cue, and in these cases the only option is to turn inward and mentally prepare to respond appropriately at the right time. And even when an external aid is possible, practitioners of the memory arts may elect to forgo it and accept the challenge of relying on their own mnemonic skills to remember the task. Here are three techniques that can substantially improve the odds.

Improving Prospective Memory by Mental Preparation

The approaches can be encoded by the acronym **ICE: I**mplementation Intentions, **C**ue Imagery, **E**xaggerated Importance. Each technique approaches the task of improving prospective memory from a different angle. The first two increase the odds of a spontaneous retrieval, while the third encourages active monitoring. We will discuss them in order of their research support beginning with the most supported. However, this says more about which ones researchers have chosen to study rather than which method is the best. If you intend to try mental techniques for improving prospective memory, I recommend experimenting with them all to find what works best for you. Students in my memory classes develop definite preferences and, surprisingly to me, there is no hands-down favorite; the first two methods are about tied in popularity. The third, while less preferred, also has its fans.

Implementation Intentions

This approach sounds almost too good to be true. If you don't want to forget to take your vitamin pill, say to yourself—and really mean it—"When I sit down at the table for breakfast tomorrow, I will take my vitamin pill." That's it. This simple act will give a major boost to your chances of taking the pill. But it's crucial that you identify both when and where the action will occur. It won't do to just say, "I will take my vitamin tomorrow," or even "I will take my vitamin at breakfast." The intention has to be super-specific about when and where this will happen.

Although memory experts have recommended this approach in the past, it was psychologist Peter Gollwitzer who developed a theoretical rationale for the implementation intention and carried out seminal studies showing its potential. It now has solid support as a helpful way to strengthen prospective memory. Just how an implementation intention works its magic is still under active investigation, but one of its contributions is creating an association between a situation and an action, such as: Sit for breakfast → Take vitamin pill. The association establishes a cue for spontaneous retrieval of the intention. That is why specificity turns out to be the key. Saying "I will take the pill in the morning" leaves open just when in the morning this is supposed to happen. An implementation intention makes the connection between the action and the trigger cue crystal clear. Implementation intentions are especially helpful when the cue for the intended action is not likely to draw attention—perhaps you want to charge your cell phone when you get home so it will be ready by the time you leave for dinner, and you worry that you won't encounter anything to remind you to do it. An implementation intention can improve the odds this will happen.

They also appear to provide added benefit for older people by compensating for age-related declines in attention and top-down control.

Here are examples of successful efforts by college students. Notice that each ends with exclamation marks to signify the serious commitment that's so necessary. The desired action must be a goal you really want to happen to fully empower an implementation intention. Half-hearted intentions don't work.

> "When I turn off the alarm in the morning, I will reset the time to 7:45 for my wife!!"
>
> "When I finish putting the evening dishes in the dishwasher, I will reply to my friend's email!!"
>
> "After we have lunch and as we are walking out of the restaurant, I will get Danielle's stuff out of my car and give it to her!!"
>
> "When the Ellen DeGeneres show is over, I will pay the bills!!"

Some fine points about implementation intentions still haven't been worked out. Does it help to make the intention out loud rather than silently? Should you repeat the intention several times when you make it? Should you imagine yourself doing the actions? Different researchers have tried these variations, but there still is no clear winner. My recommendation is to experiment to see what works for you. I find that revisiting my implementation intentions once or twice during the day increases their power.

Prospective memory isn't the only area where this method has proved useful—it also helps in many self-control situations. For example, sometimes the problem is not memory but simple inertia: you may remember that you planned to exercise this morning but just don't do it. Or you may get derailed by a competing activity: as you head out to the gym, you fall into a conversation with a neighbor. Implementation intentions can help you overcome these obstacles. They've been shown to work for a wide range of activities—exercise, healthy eating, academic achievement, taking medications, monitoring glucose, and performing breast exams.

Another application of the technique is a retention intention, one of the Dragon Principles. This involves creating a specific plan to retain memory information in a specific situation and being serious about it. In the last chapter, we saw the importance of a retention intention in learning names—once you commit to getting a name and have a plan for doing it, the chances of successful remembering shoot up.

Cue Imagery

This technique has the same goal as an implementation intention—to trigger a memory for the intended action—but it goes about it very differently. In a sense, it is everything the previous method is not. Where an implementation intention is scripted, precise, and verbal, cue imagery is ad hoc, creative, and visual. It is an approach more in keeping with the traditional memory arts.

Here's an example. To improve your chances of remembering to stop at the store for toothpaste on your way home, you might pause after you park in the morning to visualize your steering wheel smeared with globs of toothpaste and think about how unpleasant it would be to drive home with such a mess. The idea is that you will be like Pavlov's dog: when you return to the car and see the steering wheel, you will think "toothpaste!"

Unlike an implementation intention, this strategy doesn't address the plan of action. The cue simply alerts you that there is something you intend to do involving toothpaste, and it can do this in one of two ways. One possibility is that the cue will cause you to recall a clear image of a messy steering wheel when you get back in the car, but other times the cue effect can be more subtle, like an odd feeling that there is unfinished business, just enough to prompt you to search your memory for the planned action.

Here are examples of cue imagery from college students.

> "I needed to go to a craft store to buy a paper shredder before my fifty percent coupon expired, so I imagined shredded paper leading from my front door to my car with a floating paper shredder above spewing out the paper. It worked."
> "I had been forgetting to take some plastic bags to the recyclers, so I imagined a bunch of plastic bags tied to the back of my boyfriend's car and dragging like a tail. When he picked me up, I remembered."

Note how both of these examples associated the cue imagery with stimuli that were sure to be noticed in these situations. This is important—the cuing stimulus should be in focal attention. It is also important to make the images vivid and distinctive. Another good addition is giving the association extra zip with an emotional overtone. The image of toothpaste on the steering wheel adds a "yuck" factor to the cue, giving it emotional as well as visual properties. Here are two successful examples of putting emotional oomph into a cue.

"I needed to pick up my chem lab report, so I imagined a huge beaker of bubbling, dangerous acid in my backpack that needed to be carried carefully. After class when I picked up my backpack, I remembered the report."

"I had to pick up diapers from the store on my way home. I imagined I put a disgusting pile of dirty diapers on the passenger seat. When I got in the car, I thought of the diapers."

The cue imagery strategy has seen less research than implementation intentions, but Einstein and McDaniel report that participants in prospective memory studies increased their success rate by adding imaginary cues. This has been true in my own experience, as well as for students in my memory classes. To get the most out of your cues, create them at the spot where you later want them to trigger the memory. That's why I suggested you devise the toothpaste cue while you sit in the driver's seat rather than at home before the trip. Rehearsing the cue once or twice during the day will also increase its strength.

Exaggerated Importance

Highly important actions are easier to remember because their significance keeps them coming back into consciousness. Imagine you've won the lottery for a large sum of money and need to call the lottery office at ten o'clock on Wednesday to arrange to get the check. Do you think you will need a sticky note on your refrigerator for this? Not likely. The task is so important that it will remain on your mind as an active goal almost constantly. When a task becomes very important, people adopt active monitoring to detect the cue. This takes more effort, but an important task merits it. And the more important the task, the better the active monitoring becomes.

The exaggerated importance strategy tries to turn mundane tasks into super-important endeavors so that active monitoring will kick in at a high level to keep you alert for when you need to perform the action. But how can a routine task like stopping to buy toothpaste be turned into a big deal, a goal so important it will lead to active monitoring? What you need is a bold approach with plenty of imagination—you must fabricate and accept bogus reasons that this is a pressing necessity. So, you might imagine that, at this very minute, hordes of bacteria are destroying several of your teeth, and the only hope of saving them is to buy toothpaste and brush ferociously when you get home. You might even imagine you can feel them working away in your mouth. You could tell yourself that it has to be done today or the teeth will be lost, leaving gaping holes in your smile. Your goal is to turn the intended task into an activity so crucial it prompts active monitoring until it's complete. The difference between this approach and cue imagery is that the imagery here isn't tied to a focal cue intended to prompt spontaneous retrieval. Instead, the effort is aimed at the motivation for the action and tries to make it so strong that active monitoring occurs.

This is not for everyone, and it's not for every prospective memory situation, but I've found that it can be used successfully by imaginative types who enjoy a creative challenge and have enough of a theatrical flair to turn an ordinary prospective memory task into an urgent, dramatic scenario. When everything comes together, it is an interesting, fun way to get a task done. Here are two successful applications from college students, one of whom may have gone too far.

> "I was supposed to get cookies. I convinced myself that the entire world would starve to death if this didn't happen, and it became my job to save mankind. It worked. I felt like a super hero when I bought the Oreos. I get a smile on my face when I buy cookies now."

> "I needed cat food. I have four cats; two are huge. I imagined that if I didn't get the food immediately, the smaller ones would become frail and sickly while the bigger ones would become mean and voraciously try to eat me. This worked too well. I could not get cat food off my mind all day. Then I had a nightmare about it that night!"

Performing an Action at a Specified Time

When you have to do something at a specified time, like "call the plumber at four o'clock," the trigger for the action can be very slippery. Typically, you're reduced to actively monitoring the time by checking it periodically as the hour draws close. If your attention lapses, as it easily can, you will miss the cue.

One solution is to enlist an external cue, such as setting a cell phone alarm or a kitchen timer. But where is the glory for the practitioner of the memory arts in that? In fact, you can create a workable internal cue if you know where you will be and what you will be doing at about the specified time. Let's say that shortly before 4:00 P.M. you expect to get out of a staff meeting and go back to your desk. You could create a plumbing-related image that involves items in your focal attention at that time—say, an image of a backed-up drain flooding the desk and damaging your computer with foul material. Creating imagery to trigger spontaneous retrieval may not eliminate active monitoring completely, but it will improve your chances of monitoring at the right time and remembering to make the call.

A Final Thought

Prospective memory situations can offer challenges for practitioners of the memory arts that lead to satisfying successes and humbling defeats. When the costs of forgetting are not too high, why not try mental preparation techniques instead of wearing your watch backward or papering your walls with sticky notes? An added bonus is that all three of the **ICE** methods exercise basic skills of the memory arts.

In fact, you can hone your skills by creating prospective memory tasks just for that purpose. Instead of taking out the trash now, use one of the **ICE** strategies to remember to do it after you pay the bills. If you notice that a plant needs watering, why not see if you can remember to do it after you return from the store? Self-generated assignments like these—and you won't have trouble coming up with many more—allow you to practice the memory arts and experiment with different mnemonic techniques. Your successes can lead to feelings of accomplishment and build confidence in your memory. As always, pay attention to failures to see if you can understand what went wrong and learn from it.

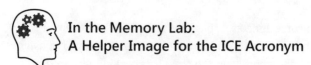

In the Memory Lab:
A Helper Image for the ICE Acronym

In this installment of the Memory Lab, I introduce the helper image for the acronym **ICE** shown on the facing page. Of course, this is a simple mnemonic, and it could function well without a helper image. I offer it primarily because I want a visual image for this chapter, just as a visual image has been associated with each of the previous chapters.

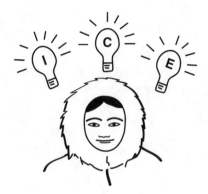

They will come into play again later when we explore memory palaces in Chapter 14. I will show you how to create a palace that will serve as a memory structure for these images and hold key points from each chapter. It will give you a compendium of important ideas from the book and place them at your mental fingertips. The Eskimo image and its association with **ICE** has a reserved spot in that memory palace.

This image has a feature that deserves mention. Recall that the purpose of a helper image is to speed the retrieval of a verbal mnemonic. The Dragon and the Friendly Llama helper images cued the first words in their associated acrostics—"Romantic dragons . . . " and "Friendly llamas . . . ". Interestingly, the Eskimo image for **ICE** does more than just prompt the acronym—the light bulbs suggest an intention popping into mind. For me, this is an ideal helper image because the "light coming on" is associated with the kind of situation where the mnemonic is relevant, one requiring prospective memory, and the Eskimo helps launch a verbal mnemonic for dealing with it. These cues have the potential to work together and rapidly bring the mnemonic to mind.

9

Remembering Facts

New facts enter our lives from every direction. Tomorrow's weather forecast, the latest political scandal, revised dietary guidelines, an online story about a raging forest fire. Most of these factoids will never play a useful role in our lives, and we will eventually forget them. This is as it should be. The memory system is fine-tuned to retain useful information, and most of the day's new facts won't make the cut. Although it is true that we sometimes remember the oddest things—like how fast a cheetah can run or a line from an old movie—these are exceptions. Most facts that we don't use in some way will be lost to us.

Interestingly, though, it's also true that important facts sometimes suffer the same fate. This might be because we don't use them immediately, like what you should do if your child suffers an asthma attack. Or it might be the sheer quantity of facts you are facing, like a biology test next week or new procedures required for your job. The good news, as we will see in this chapter, is that there are smart, efficient ways to retain demanding new facts in situations where they would otherwise be forgotten.

Before we turn to these strategies, let's consider what happens to newly learned facts if we do nothing to enhance retention. More than seventy years ago, psychologist Herbert Spitzer carried out a classic study of the forgetting process as part of his doctoral dissertation at the State University of Iowa. He asked 3,605 sixth-grade children in ninety-one Iowa schools to read short, factual essays on neutral topics. The large number of children meant he could divide them into groups and test each group after a different period of time to map out how the children retained the material over a sixty-three-day period.

Spitzer gave each child a surprise multiple-choice test so that different children were tested after 0, 1, 7, 14, 21, 28, and 63 days. The results plotted on the graph below show how forgetting takes place with the passage of time. Notice the shape of the curve—many details faded shortly after the children learned them, while others were lost more gradually as time passed. This is what happens to forgettable information that is not put to use.

Facts can have various forgetting curves. Their shapes are usually similar to the one Spitzer found, but the time frame might be sped up or slowed down. When new information is especially difficult—say, the new Japanese vocabulary words you just learned—the time period for the forgetting curve might well be in hours rather than days. On the other hand, the details of a friend's birthday party could have a forgetting curve with the same shape as Spitzer's spread over months rather than days.

The Dragon Principles and the specialized mnemonics we have seen in previous chapters are ways to combat forgetting. Here we expand our options by looking more closely at memory practice, the Dragon Principle that strengthens a memory by rehearsing it. Memory practice has long been known to be a powerful, reliable way to enhance memory for facts, and a flurry of recent research has clarified how best to apply it.

Memory Practice Options

Let's say you've just acquired a new and forgettable fact: the name of the Greek goddess of memory, Mnemosyne. The diagram on the next page

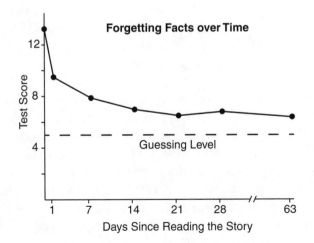

Three Ways to Strengthen Memory for a Greek Goddess

Recall
    Her name is _____

Recognition
    Her name is:
        (a) Memoria
        (b) Mnemosyne
        (c) Mabel

Restudy
    Her name is Mnemosyne

---

shows three different ways to apply memory practice to refresh and strengthen your memory for her name.

> *Recall.* The most straightforward way is to recall it. This is the way we learn many of the facts we have at our fingertips—our friends' names, our partner's birthday, the PIN for the ATM. Each time we recall facts like these, memory is strengthened, and over time it becomes rock solid.
>
> *Recognition.* This form of memory practice is used by students who study for their SAT or MCAT tests by taking practice multiple-choice tests. Fact memory is strengthened when they recognize a correct answer.
>
> *Restudying.* In the third approach, memory is freshened by restudying the material. Think of the speaker who looks over her notes one last time before walking to the podium.

When memory scientists investigate the effectiveness of these methods, they find that the best approach depends on how soon people are tested after they practice—the method that works best when the test is immediate is not best when the test is delayed. This was the conclusion of a study by Washington University researchers Henry Roediger and Jeffrey Karpicke, who compared the recall method to the restudying method. They asked college students to read passages on topics such as sea otters. After they finished reading, the researchers gave them additional time to study for a future test, either by going back over the material several times (the restudying approach) or by trying to recall what they could remember of it (the recall approach). Next the researchers divided the students into groups and tested them after different periods of time—some after five minutes, others after either two days or a week.

The results are shown in the bar graph below. When the test occurred only five minutes after finishing the exercise, restudying led to higher memory scores than recall. But when the test was delayed for two days or a week, the recall method became increasingly superior. After a week, the students who practiced their memories using recall remembered thirty-eight percent more than those who restudied. Studies with even longer retention periods have shown that recall continues to shine as the preferred rehearsal strategy in all delayed memory tests.

What about recognition? Multiple-choice tests are a useful way to strengthen memory—their benefits are similar to recall. But in head-to-head comparisons, the recall method is usually better; and a recall test doesn't carry the risk that you will learn wrong information by remembering an incorrect answer, as can happen in multiple-choice recognition tests.

Repeated Memory Practice

Roediger and Karpicke allowed their students only one memory practice session, but most realistic situations will demand more. Remembering the

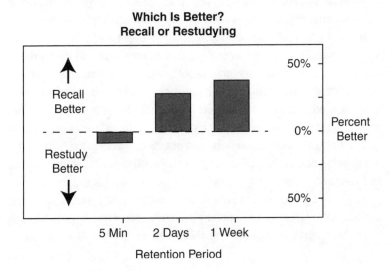

name "Mnemosyne," even for a few weeks, will probably require that you practice it several times. Just how that practice is carried out turns out to be every bit as important as which type of memory practice you use. Say you decide to practice Mnemosyne's name five times. You then have to decide whether you will carry out the practice in one sitting or spread it out over five practice sessions. When I introduced memory practice in Chapter 4, I suggested spacing practice out, and I offered Dominic O'Brien's Rule of Five as one way to do it: practice the memory after an hour, a day, a week, two weeks, and a month. I'll have more to say about spacing rules like this shortly, but before I get to that, consider the alternative of concentrating all the practice into one session.

This is the way some students study for a test—an intense study session in which they restudy their textbooks and notes over and over until they feel they know the material. This is "cramming," of course, the primary studying method used by between twenty-five and fifty percent of college students. Psychologists call this form of memory rehearsal "massed" because all the practice takes place in one session. It yields good memory performance in the short run and has saved many a student from a bad grade. But it has a serious drawback: the memory boost it provides is short lived, and students are likely to find a week after the exam that they can no longer remember many of the facts they crammed into their heads. It is an unfortunate truth that massed practice leads to poor long-term retention.

This brings me to a major point about memory practice: the best way to pump up memory for facts depends on the situation, as summarized in the box on the facing page. Do you need facts at your fingertips for a looming, one-shot event such as next week's conference presentation? Then do your final preparation within hours of the event and practice the material by reviewing it over and over until it is firmly in mind. Using the restudy method like this takes less mental effort than practicing by memory recall and yields stronger immediate memory gains. But you need to do this with full knowledge that the facts you master will be yours only temporarily—forgetting will likely be fast and extensive. If the information is valuable for the future, then it is much better to practice the relevant facts by recalling them using one of the self-testing methods I'll describe shortly and to space out the practice sessions. This is the way to build lasting memories.

These two strategies are certainly not mutually exclusive, and in practical situations like an important presentation, it makes sense to prepare early in several sessions using the recall method with self-testing. Then

Memory Practice Recommendations

Near-Term Use (hours)	Longer-Term Use (days and more)
Restudy with Massed Repetitions	Recall with Spaced Repetitions

plan a mini-cram session shortly before the big moment, with an emphasis on rereading the material rather than recalling it. This sets the stage for a solid performance now and good retention later. This is also how good students get the most out of college courses, with both good grades on tests and lasting knowledge.

Why Is Spaced Memory Recall Effective?

Robert Bjork, a UCLA memory scientist, proposed that the benefit of spaced retrieval practice comes from the forgetting that occurs between practice sessions. If you wait to practice recalling Mnemosyne's name until tomorrow, it won't be as fresh as it is now and will require some mental effort to remember. It is that effort, Bjork says, that benefits memory. He calls it "desirable difficulty," and it appears to be an essential requirement to achieve long-term memory benefit from retrieval practice. If a memory is still easily recallable, there is little gain in practicing it, but if you have to work a bit to retrieve it, you will build long-lasting memory strength.

The concept of desirable difficulty explains why recall is superior to restudying when it comes to building memory strength. When you recall a memory, as in "The Greek goddess's name is _____," you expend effort to retrieve it, and this translates into greater memory strength for the future. But when you reread the same fact, as in "Her name is Mnemosyne," you refresh the memory all right, but there is less mental effort involved and therefore less enduring memory improvement takes place.

So, how much difficulty is desirable? If we are talking about maximizing long-term memory strength, then the more difficulty the better, even if you wait so long to rehearse the memory that you may not be able to recall it at all and have to relearn it. An experience like this will likely benefit the memory more in the long run than a comparable recall experience at shorter spacing with less difficulty, one where you successfully remember the material. That said, relearning facts is an irritation I can do without, and I prefer not to wait so long to practice a fact that I stumble and can't recall it. The Rule of Five is an example of putting this philosophy into action. The idea is to start memory practice shortly after learning a fact, when the memory can still be recalled, and follow up with additional practice using ever longer spacing intervals as the memory becomes stronger. Bjork and his colleague Thomas Landauer call this approach "expanding retrieval practice." When you choose your spacing adjustments well, you'll experience desirable difficulty with few memory failures. This leaves you feeling positive and confident in your memory and not humbled by a failure. Professional mnemonists endorse this approach.

The memory material you want to retain is the best guide for using expanding retrieval practice. Suppose you want a more secure password for your online banking account, and following the bank's recommendations for a super-safe password, you come up with kRm-3bY. This will be challenging to remember, and you will definitely need spaced practice if you want to hold on to it. That first rehearsal after the initial learning is particularly important, because early forgetting can be so rapid—we saw this in Spitzer's forgetting curve. Getting the new memory through this highly vulnerable period needs to be a priority. But desirable difficulty is important even in this early practice. If the first recall attempt is too soon, the memory will come to mind so readily there will be little benefit. Wait too long, though, and your pride will suffer when you find you can't remember.

This is a Goldilocks situation—you want enough desirable difficulty, but not too much. It's easy to tell when you've waited too long to rehearse because recall fails. But how do you tell that you've waited long enough? Here is a practical way to judge it. Pay attention to the lag between the moment you search for the memory and the moment it comes to mind. If you can detect a lag, even a small one, it means your system had to work to retrieve the memory. You might experience this as "the password is . . . ah . . . kRm-3bY." Take that as a sign you've met the requirement for desirable difficulty. And if the retrieval required you to search hard for the memory, so much the better.

The concept of desirable difficulty shows why the Rule of Five is a rule of thumb and not a hard-and-fast prescription. It is best used as a starting point that you can adjust depending on the kind of material and the length of time it is to be retained. When the material is difficult, like this password, tighten up the spacing. If the material is easy, relax the spacing. When you need to retain it for a long time, five times may not be enough.

Why Isn't Spaced Retrieval Practice Used More Commonly?

Despite the clear superiority of the recall method over the restudy method, students report they rarely use it when they study. One reason is that it is simply more work to practice facts by arranging a self-test and recalling them. But there is also something else going on. Studying by recalling just doesn't seem as effective to students as reading back through their notes. Suppose we ask college students to respond to this scenario:

Students in two different classes read the same one-page essay. In Class A, the students were asked to write down as much as they could remember after they finished. In Class B, the students were given an opportunity to restudy the passage after they finished. After one week, all students were tested on their memory for the passage. Which class would you expect to have the higher test scores?

(a) Class A   (b) Class B

When memory researcher Jennifer McCabe posed a similar question to college students, she found an overwhelming preference for the second strategy, restudying, even though this approach is known to be inferior to the recall method in this situation. Why did the students get it wrong? Most likely, they based their answers on their own experience. They knew that when they finished reading material over and over, they felt confident in their memory. The facts seemed clear and fresh. They popped into mind quickly and easily as the students reviewed them. This is not always so when recalling facts in a self-test—more effort is often required to bring the facts to mind, so they don't seem as solid. From a student's point of view, it can seem obvious which method—restudying—produces better learning. Robert Bjork refers to this as an "illusion of competence" after restudying. The student concludes that she knows the material well based on the confident mastery she feels at that moment. And she expects that the same mastery will be there several days later when the exam takes place. But this is unlikely. The same illusion of competence is at work during cramming, when the facts feel secure and firmly grasped. While that is indeed true at the time, it's a mistake to assume that long-lasting memory strength has been created.

Illusions of competence are seductive. They can easily mislead people into misjudging the strength of their memory, and they can encourage students to adopt study methods that undermine long-term retention. The best defense is to use proven memory techniques and to be leery of making predictions about future memory strength based on how solid the memory seems right now.

Harnessing the Power of Retrieval Practice

Retrieval practice should always be in the picture when you need to retain difficult factual material for anything other than immediate use. Mnemonics can reduce the amount of practice you need—often dramatically—but even with good mnemonics, some retrieval practice will be helpful. Here are several approaches.

Read–Rehearse–Review

Just one round of practice can help clarify difficult material and make it easier to hang on to it. For example, if a news story you are reading describes two opposing arguments about reducing Pentagon spending, you can make sure you have them solidly in memory by giving yourself an impromptu self-test. All it takes is to pause after the passage, recall the material, check its accuracy, and then move on. Researcher Mark McDaniel and his collaborators demonstrated the benefits of a quick self-test by asking college students to do exactly that. They read a passage, then said out loud as much as they could remember before reviewing the passage again as a check. The researchers found that memory for the material was superior to that of other students who either read the passage twice or took notes on their reading. Pausing for a self-test after a tricky but important passage is a simple but effective way to improve memory for that material.

Share with Others

Another way to strengthen memory for facts is to talk about them with others. Microsoft founder and philanthropist Bill Gates is a voracious reader with wide-ranging interests. In a television interview, he described how he often discusses the material with his wife, Melinda. He also maintains a blog where he reviews and comments on books he reads. These sharing activities are rewarding, and they allow him to retrieve and strengthen ideas he finds provocative, setting the stage for lasting memories.

Self-Testing

Bill Gates notwithstanding, if you are facing a challenging biology test next week, or you are trying to master new procedures for your job, you will need a more systematic approach, and it should include spaced retrieval practice. An effective strategy is to use a form of self-testing that presents a cue, allows you to recall a fact, and then provides feedback on your answer. Textbook study questions or practice tests can provide this, but by far the most popular student self-testing strategy is flashcards—one survey found that two-thirds of students used them. And it's not just college students. The market for commercially produced flashcards is large and lucrative, judging from the offerings available online. There are flashcards to help toddlers learn colors and shapes; flashcards to teach multiplication and division; flashcards to master chemistry, history, literature, and psychology; flashcards for the SAT, GRE, MCAT, and other major exams. Competing with paper versions of flashcards are electronic versions that move the self-testing online. Flashcards—either written or electronic—create almost ideal conditions for self-testing: You read a memory cue, try to recall the information, and check the answer.

You might worry that retrieval practice of this kind would produce only narrow, rote learning, but the evidence doesn't support this concern. In fact, self-testing is associated with a range of desirable educational outcomes. It not only helps memory for the facts tested but also provides a boost for related facts. With more retrieval practice, students become better able to apply the facts to new situations, and they can more easily learn related knowledge. For example, researchers at Washington University taught a group of students how to classify birds as finches, orioles, swallows, and other avian families using an electronic version of flashcards. Other students studied the birds and their classifications the same number of times without recalling their own answer first. Those who used retrieval practice not only were able to classify the birds they studied more accurately; they were also better at guessing the proper classification for birds they had never seen before.

The SCRR Method

This technique adapts the flashcard method for use with printed material of all sorts without the need to prepare special cards. It allows you to quickly set up conditions for self-testing. The acronym **SCRR** gives its essential steps.

Segment: divide the material into key ideas.
Cue: create a cue for each idea.
Retrieve: use the cues to recall the ideas.
Review: check the accuracy of the memory.

To show this method at work, I have applied it to the passage shown on the facing page. First, I identified the key points in the text worthy of expending effort to retain. Underlining or highlighting is my preference, and I've done so in the passage. The more focused and restrained I can make my marking, the easier it will be to zero in on what's really useful. Next I examined what I marked and segmented the material into major ideas by adding horizontal lines out into the margin. It's important to be selective here, because not all of the text will have ideas that deserve to be remembered. What you're looking for are facts so important that they justify the work it will take to retain them. I marked the first section of text with an "X," a signal to skip it, because it didn't pass this test. I then found two major ideas in the rest of the passage and marked the segments. I created a memory cue for each and wrote it in the margin. The cue can be a word, a phrase, or even a drawing—anything relevant to the concept, just enough to suggest it but not enough to give it away. Each segment becomes the equivalent of a flashcard, and the cue word is equivalent to what would be on the front side.

With the cues in place, the first self-test can begin by covering the passage to expose only the cues and then recalling the relevant facts. The final step is to review the information. This should wait until you have responded to all the cues, because there is a memory benefit to delaying the review step a bit. But the review step should not be skipped—studies show that feedback of this kind adds to the effectiveness of self-testing.

How Many Self-Tests?

Self-testing should be repeated until you have thoroughly mastered the information. At the very least, continue the self-testing until you can make

Segmenting and cuing a previously underlined text

Education is about more than memory, of course, but the need to acquire and remember course content is an inescapable requirement. Not only is memory required to survive tests, but students who acquire a solid knowledge base are in a good position to leverage it into other successes. Critical thinking, creativity, problem solving and technical competence, all valued educational outcomes, draw on knowledge previously learned and remembered through activities carried out in study sessions.

The first point to make about studying is that the amount of time students devote to it has a surprisingly poor relationship to academic success. Many college students with mediocre grades study just as much as top students, but they don't get the same benefit. While intellectual differences among students are involved, they are far from an explanation of what's going on. A considerable body of data suggests that students are often seriously short changed in what they get from their studying. This is a costly lost opportunity, and improvements are worthy of effort.

studying & success

A study session can have either of two quite different goals: learning new factual knowledge or learning a new skill. The first situation is associated with content courses like history, biology or psychology where a significant body of factual knowledge must be mastered from lectures and textbooks. The second situation arises in courses like English composition, mathematics or computer programming where the student is expected to produce a product or solve a problem. While factual knowledge is necessary to meet these requirements, it is not enough. Competent performance in skill-based courses requires procedural knowledge that can only be acquired by experience.

Two kinds of courses

one perfect pass through the cue words and there is evidence that three perfect passes may be better. This applies regardless of whether you are using traditional flashcards or the SCRR method.

After the initial learning, you can decide how much more spaced practice you will need, and this depends on how long you want to retain the information. In a study of remembering detailed academic information, five additional rehearsals spaced a week apart led to sixty-three percent retention one month later and forty-eight percent retention at four months. The Rule of Five using the spacing of an hour, a day, a week, two weeks, and a month should produce generally similar results for this kind of material. Better retention would require more rehearsal.

Organizing Facts

I find that arranging facts into an organizational structure is an aid to memory practice because it helps connect the facts. I prefer a visual approach called "mind mapping," a technique advocated by British memory trainer Tony Buzan. The available research shows that mapping is itself an aid to memory, but I find a special benefit when using mapping with retrieval practice. To illustrate it, I created the map below depicting key facts in this chapter. I started by placing the central topic, "Retaining facts," in the center, and then I added a radial line for each major theme. As each line moved outward, I added branches to identify important concepts. Buzan recommends embellishing the mind map with drawings, colors, and flourishes to make it more memorable.

To use the mind map for memory practice, treat the entries as memory cues and recall details about them. Follow this with a quick review of the material to check for accuracy. When the map is not too complex, you may find that you can remember the map itself without needing to refer to a paper copy. This allows you to practice both the organization and the specific information.

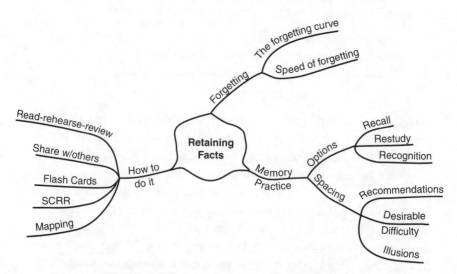

A memory map of key ideas presented in this chapter.

The Permastore

We retain some facts for long periods. Think back to your high school history or geography or science classes. If you take a minute, you will almost certainly find bits and pieces of information from these classes that you haven't retrieved for years. Ohio Wesleyan University researcher Harry Bahrick calls this repository of long-lasting information the "permastore"—information that seems to have escaped the forgetting process.

Bahrick arrived at the idea of the permastore while studying long-term memory for information learned in college Spanish classes. He recruited about 600 Wesleyan graduates who had been out of school from a few months to fifty years. It turned out that most had used Spanish little if at all in the intervening years, and this allowed him to examine how that learning held up over time. The results of Spanish–English vocabulary tests he gave them are plotted in the graph below.

Look first at the findings for multiple-choice tests, and notice how they stabilize at around seventy percent of what students score right after their last Spanish course. What is eye-popping is that the line stays relatively

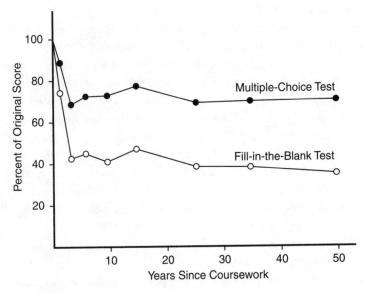

The results of Spanish vocabulary tests taken by university alumni who studied Spanish as undergraduates.

flat for fifty years, a remarkable period of stable knowledge. When students are required to actually recall the answer instead of recognizing it, performance is lower, but there is the same period of flat retention. The differences between the two curves show that permastore memories vary in strength. The multiple-choice test can pick up knowledge that's not strong enough to be remembered in a recall test—for example, a student might correctly choose "redhead" as the meaning of *pelirrojo* when it is offered as an option but not be able to come up with it independently.

What permastore memories have in common is their stability—forgetting appears to be suspended for these memories. Bahrick's discovery of the permastore was quite unexpected. Since his groundbreaking work, additional evidence has given the concept solid support. Similar long-lasting memories have been found for mathematics knowledge, street names of childhood neighborhoods, and high school classmates.

How do facts escape forgetting and become part of the permastore? Bahrick combed through his large sample to see what student characteristics were associated with the number of memories in their permastores. Two major predictors emerged. First was the level of initial learning. Students who received an "A" in their Spanish courses often performed fifty percent better on Bahrick's tests than students who scored a "C." Stronger initial learning had helped move more knowledge into the permastore. The second factor was the number of Spanish courses students took. Each additional course not only taught the students new information but also provided an opportunity to practice what they had learned in previous courses—foreign language classes, unlike many academic subjects, provide opportunities for spaced retrieval practice of previously learned material. This added practice shows up in the permastore. Other settings with regular practice opportunities also show substantial permastore knowledge. One dramatic example is memory for high school classmates. Bahrick found that people could match yearbook pictures to the names of their classmates with almost ninety percent accuracy even after thirty-five years. He attributes this impressive retention to the opportunities for memory practice throughout the high school years.

Bahrick's retention curves show that most forgetting occurs during the first several years as weaker memories drop out. He believes that once memories survive the first three to five years, they have permastore status and can be stable for decades. The take-home message from Bahrick's extensive work is that solid initial learning coupled with spaced retrieval practice can allow new facts to get through this crucial period and become remarkably durable memories.

A Final Thought

When important facts need help to stay memorable, the practitioner of the memory arts has two options. The first is to improve the encoding of the facts in memory. This is always a useful place to start, and we have seen a variety of ways to do it, beginning with the Dragon Principles. Once the memory is established, the second option can come into play—strengthen retention with memory practice. The two options are complementary and offer powerful ways to combat forgetting and sometimes even add to the permastore.

 **In the Memory Lab:
Rhymes as Memory Aids**

Rhymes have long been used as memory aids. I'll have more to say about both rhyme and rhythm in Chapter 13. My purpose here is to invite you to try out two rhyming mnemonics to gain experience with this approach.

First, consider a rhyme extolling the virtues of spaced retrieval practice:

Henry

*There once was a boy named Henry
Who tried to improve his memory.
He practiced the facts he faced
With retrieval well spaced,
And found his recall exemplary.*

Here is a second rhyme to help retain the SCRR method:

*Segment, Cue
Retrieve, Review*

When you practice recalling the rhymes, try exaggerating them in a rhythmic way, such as, "There ONCE was a boy named HENRY / who TRIED to improve his MEMORY / . . . " You will find that an exaggerated rhythm makes the rhymes easier to remember.

A visual mnemonic is useful here, and my suggestion appears below. It shows memory cues organized on a cartoon image of Henry, who displays an "H" (a cue for the Henry limerick) and an octagon to suggest a "stop" sign (a cue for the "s" sound of "segment," the first word of SCRR). I also added a dumbbell to the image to suggest the connection between the Rule of Five and Desirable Difficulty when it comes to increasing memory strength. To retain the information cued by the Henry image, you will need to practice recalling it. Consider designing a rehearsal schedule and evaluating how well it works.

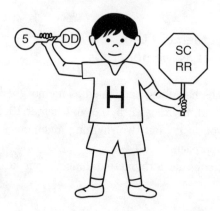

A mnemonic for ways to improve memory for facts.

10

Remembering Numbers

On November 20, 2005, Chao Lu, a twenty-three-year-old resident of Yangling, China, recited the first 61,890 digits of the mathematical constant *pi* from memory, surpassing a previous record and earning him a place in the *Guinness Book of World Records*. It is a record he continues to hold as this is written.

Chao Lu was inspired by the fact that a Japanese man held the record for memorizing *pi* prior to his attempt, a fact that didn't sit well with him. "It was Zu Chongzhi, the ancient Chinese mathematician, who discovered the ratio between the circumference to the diameter of the circle," he said, "and Chinese should win the *pi* recitation contest." He began serious training for the record in 2004, working three to five hours a day, sometimes as many as ten. He estimated his preparation time during that last year at 1,300 hours. It was arduous—he was plagued by insomnia, discouragement, and even hair loss.

Chao Lu planned to recite 90,000 digits when he began the record attempt, a process that required clearly announcing one digit after another in the presence of judges. This too was grueling. According to the Guinness rules, no more than fifteen seconds can elapse between saying successive digits, so food and bathroom breaks are not possible. After twenty-four hours and four minutes, on digit number 67,891, he mistakenly said "five" instead of "zero," ending his attempt and establishing the current record.

One of the most fascinating—and astonishing—aspects of his triumph is that Chao Lu does not have unusual memory abilities. Several years after setting the record, when he was twenty-seven, he cooperated with Chinese and American psychologists by taking a battery of memory tests involving both numbers and words. Their conclusion was that his native abilities were squarely within the normal range. His remarkable accomplishment was the result of mnemonic technique and hard work.

Chao Lu's record impresses not only because of the quantity of what he retained but also because his achievement involved numbers, memory material that seems especially forgettable. Numbers are bland, abstract, and unremarkable. The mathematical constant *pi* is a perfect source for someone seeking an unending supply of meaningless digits because it can be calculated out to as many decimal places as you like. The only practical way to retain the digits is to rely on mnemonic techniques. In this chapter we will see a variety of ways to remember numbers, ranging from the simple to the sophisticated, including the system used by Chao Lu.

But before we get to that, you may ask why anyone should bother learning ways to remember numbers. I assume that you, like me, have not the slightest interest in challenging Chao Lu's record. Nowadays it is seldom necessary to store numbers in your own memory. Phone numbers, catalog numbers, addresses, complete with maps to get you there, are all saved for us on electronic devices. And you can jot down the occasional number you must retain on a scrap of paper or record it on your cell phone.

So what advantage does remembering numbers convey? We know that mnemonic techniques for other material have practical utility—they can sharpen your ability to remember names and facts, and they can improve your prospective memory for tasks you need to accomplish. But remembering numbers is another matter. Is spending effort to remember numbers a good investment? You must decide that for yourself, of course, but here is my take on it.

Taking the Stairs

In fact, numbers offer a practitioner of the memory arts small but rewarding challenges. You'll need only a short focused effort to hold on to most numbers. But this brief task will call into action your highest, most sophisticated mental abilities—attention, working memory, and top-down control—as you deploy a mnemonic strategy to convert a bland number into an easily remembered entity. And when you successfully recall it later, you will deservedly be pleased with yourself. This is mental exercise that you could easily avoid but that you deliberately choose to engage in. Like those who walk past the elevator and take the stairs instead, mnemonists who reject external memory aids choose to rely on their own personal resources rather than artificial assistance, and in return they get exercise they otherwise wouldn't. This is the mindset I recommend for those who would apply memory techniques to numbers: Do it for the challenge, the mental exercise, and the personal satisfaction. Let practical benefits of remembering numbers be a bonus.

How to Remember Numbers: Three Easy Ways

The key to remembering numbers is to find a way to make these ordinary objects into something concrete and memorable. Sometimes it doesn't take much to make that happen.

Find a Pattern

We usually take for granted that numbers are meaningless and we don't look closely at them. A phone number like 279-9980 can seem like just another jumble of digits, but if you try, you can sometimes discover interesting memory-enhancing features. That is the essence of the find-a-pattern approach—you really look at the number and try to find something meaningful in it.

If the number is long, it is usually best to focus on chunks of two, three, or four digits. You might discover a number sequence, 3456; or a date, 1492; or a pattern of odd or even digits, 1357; or someone's birthday, 614 → June 14; or a perfect square, 625; or a pleasing symmetric number, 383; or a mathematical relation, 257 → 2 + 5 = 7; or a family member's age, 36; or repeated digits, 4466; or a telephone area code, 206; or a familiar address, 1600.

Now let's look back at that phone number, 279-9980. Can you make anything out of it? The patterns and connections people make to numbers are highly individualistic, so there is no right or wrong answer. Here is what I found. First I noticed all the nines—not only are there three in a row, but the first two digits, 2 and 7, add up to 9. I also saw that the first three digits ascend (279) while the last four descend (9980). And I know that 9 x 9 = 81, which almost but not quite works for that second group.

With this assortment of observations in hand, what else will I need to retain the number? If I plan to use it in a few hours, I'll probably need nothing more. My associations should keep the number available to me until then. If I want to keep it longer, or if the number feels slippery, I may need to work in some rehearsal in which I think back to the patterns I found.

This approach has one more important benefit. Although finding a pattern or some other connection to the number is the goal, the deep processing involved in searching for it also has value. This means that even when you come up dry and can't find anything special about the number, you may discover that it is firmly in your memory from the serious effort you made. By focusing on the number and looking at it from all angles to find a pattern, you produce brain activation that leaves behind memory for the digits themselves.

An Acrostic for Numbers

Another way to turn a number into a meaningful entity is to use a modified version of the acrostic. In this application, the memory cue is the number of letters in each word of a sentence. Consider the PIN number 6327. You could remember it by the sentence "Prince Tom is wealthy." The length of the words gives the number—Prince (6) Tom (3) is (2) wealthy (7). Since the sentence is meaningful, it is relatively easy to retain. Here is an example especially for those who might have a use for the mathematical constant *pi*—it is a sentence that gives its value to eight digits: "How I wish I could enumerate *pi* easily" (3.1415926).

Encoding a zero is a problem for the acrostic strategy, but a workable solution is to let any word beginning with a "z" stand for zero. Thus, 3306 could be encoded "The dog zestfully played." Another problem, one without a remedy, is that not all numbers can be turned into sentences (try 9119). In most cases, though, the modified acrostic turns out to be a useful way to remember a number that you need to retain over time.

The Number–Shape System

Imagery is another way to give numbers the concrete meaning they are missing, and systems for doing this go back at least to the seventeenth century. One technique is to make use of concrete objects that have shapes somewhat similar to the shapes of specific digits.

Some possibilities along with specific examples are on the facing page.

0: Ball, wheel, world globe
1: Candle, rocket, pencil
2: Swan, sickle, duck
3: Handcuffs, double chin, breasts
4: Sail on a boat, pennant on a pole, axe
5: Seahorse, S-hook, snake
6: Golf club, elephant's trunk, cherry
7: Boomerang, cliff edge, carpenter's square
8: Snowman, hourglass, spectacles
9: Balloon on a string, tennis racket, sperm

You could use this approach to remember you left your car on the fifth floor of the parking garage by imagining a large seahorse sitting in the passenger seat. For a dental appointment on the twenty-sixth of the month at three o'clock, you could picture a swan holding a golf club in its bill and charging a dentist who is in handcuffs. The number–shape system works best with one- and two-digit numbers.

Remembering the Calendar

An application that puts the number–shape system to good use is a mental calendar. It is based on the fact that if you know the date of the first Sunday of a month, you can calculate the date and weekday of any other day in that

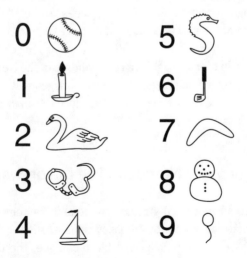

month. If you know twelve Sundays, you have a mental calendar for a year. Here's how this works. Say I want to know the day of the week my wife's birthday, August 27, falls on. Using the method I'll describe shortly, I recall that the first Sunday of August this year is August 3. Three Sundays hence is 21 + 3 = August 24, so I know her birthday will be on a Wednesday (24 + 3). Or I might want to know the date of the second Tuesday in June, when a committee I serve on meets. I know that the first Sunday of June is June 1, so I calculate that the first Tuesday is June 3 (1 + 2) and therefore the second Tuesday is June 10 (3 + 7).

To use this system, you need to have in memory the twelve Sundays in the current year. I do this by connecting an image for the month with a number–shape image for the date. The month images are matters of personal choice; here are some possibilities:

January—a New Year's baby	February—Cupid
March—a lion	April—a fool

I associate each month image with the appropriate number–shape image. For example, in 2014, the first Sunday in January is January 5, so I imagine a New Year's baby riding a seahorse. In February, the first Sunday falls on February 2, so Cupid is feeding a group of swans. With an occasional rehearsal, these images stay readily available. As with any calendar, as the year draws to an end, I have to replace it for the coming year. I keep the same month images, but I create new associations that are different from last year's using alternative number–shape cues. To help keep the images from different years separate, I select a distinctive color for the year and work it into every image. This year, all my calendar images have conspicuous red elements in them—such as a red seahorse in the New Year's image and red swans in the cupid image. Next year's images will feature blue elements. Color adds a helpful retrieval cue to reduce the chances of mixing up images from different years.

How to Remember Numbers: The Major System

Now we turn to an industrial-strength mnemonic for remembering numbers. This old and well-proven system is variously called the major system, the phonetic system, the number-syllable technique, the digit-consonant mnemonic, and the digit-to-sound system. Psychologist Allan Paivio traced its early form to 1648. Subsequent mnemonists refined it until the present version emerged in the mid-nineteenth century. This powerful technique has been endorsed by generations of mnemonists, and it is widely used in various forms by memory performers and competitors to this day.

The major system is a scheme to turn numbers into meaningful words. This is done with a code that connects specific sounds with specific numbers, a code that uses only sounds of consonants. For example, the "t" and "d" sounds represent the number "1." Vowels and unvoiced consonants carry no numeric meaning, so they can be added as necessary to create a word. This means that the number "1" can be represented in many ways: "tie," "doe," or "dough." In each case, an abstract number is transformed into a tangible, concrete entity, greatly improving its memorability. A two-digit number like "11" is represented by a word with two t/d sounds like "tot," "tide," "dad," or "duty."

Each digit is associated with specific sounds as shown in the table on the next page. Also shown are rationales for the codes that can serve as memory aids to retain them as well as the rules for how they are used.

To get a feel for the code, try decoding these two-digit numbers:

bell, coin, chef, lily

Now try your hand at finding words to represent these numbers:

41, 19, 47, 35

Three-digit representations are illustrated by these mnemonics for measurement conversions from imperial to metric units:

1 inch = 25.4 mm (kneeler)
1 mile = 1.61 km (dashed)
1 pound = 0.454 kg (roller)

In principle, any number can be recast into concrete words with this system. Memory experts Harry Lorayne and Jerry Lucas showcase the possibilities by suggesting the sentence "a beautiful naked blonde jumps up and down" to encode the twenty-digit number 9185-2719-5216-3909-2112. But, in truth, it would be the rare long number that has such a memorable representation, and even if it did, it would take a major investment of time

Number-to-Sound Conventions of the Major System

Digit	Sound	Memory Aid
0	z, s, soft c	"zero"
1	t, d	each has one down stroke
2	n	two down strokes
3	m	three down strokes
4	r	as in "four"
5	L	L is the Roman numeral for 50
6	j, sh, ch, soft g	flipping j makes it similar to a 6
7	k, q, hard c or g	imagine a k made from two 7s
8	f, v	a script f looks like an 8
9	p, b	p flips to a 9; b rotates to a 9

Number-to-Sound Rules

- Sounds not listed—vowels and h, w, or y—can be freely used to make words and carry no numeric meaning (hat is 1, woods is 10).
- When a consonant is silent, it doesn't count (lamb is 53, knife is 28).
- When a repeated consonant is pronounced as a single sound, it only counts once (mummy is 33).
- The letter x is not used.

to discover it. That's why the most common way to use the major system is to divide a long number into one- and two-digit chunks and encode each chunk using a standard set of words.

Suppose you wanted to apply the approach to that phone number: 279-9980. First you divide it into chunks: 2 + 79 + 99 + 80. Next you plug in standard words for these chunks that you have previously committed to memory—a full list of them appears in the table on the facing page. This yields: hen (2) + cop (79) + baby (99) + fuzz (80). To bind them together, you invent a story and visualize it: A **hen** dressed as a **cop** is anxiously watching over a **baby** as a cloud of **fuzz** blows by.

Major System Codes for 110 Numbers

0—zoo	12—tin	34—mower	56—leech	78—cave
1—tie	13—tomb	35—mule	57—log	79—cop
2—hen	14—tire	36—match	58—lava	80—fuzz
3—ma	15—towel	37—mug	59—lip	81—foot
4—rye	16—tissue	38—movie	60—cheese	82—fan
5—law	17—tack	39—mop	61—chute	83—foam
6—shoe	18—taffy	40—rose	62—chain	84—fur
7—cow	19—tub	41—rat	63—chum	85—filly
8—ivy	20—nose	42—rain	64—chair	86—fish
9—bee	21—net	43—ram	65—cello	87—fog
00—sauce	22—nun	44—rower	66—choo-choo	88—five
01—suit	23—name	45—roll	67—chalk	89—fob
02—sun	24—Nero	46—roach	68—chef	90—bus
03—sum	25—nail	47—rock	69—chip	91—bat
04—seer	26—notch	48—roof	70—case	92—bone
05—sail	27—neck	49—rope	71—cot	93—bum
06—sash	28—navy	50—lace	72—coin	94—bear
07—sock	29—knob	51—lad	73—comb	95—bell
08—safe	30—mouse	52—lion	74—car	96—beach
09—soap	31—mat	53—lamb	75—coal	97—book
10—toes	32—moon	54—lure	76—cage	98—beef
11—tot	33—mummy	55—lily	77—cake	99—baby

The major system is flexible enough to handle just about any situation where we need to retain a number. For example, I have a combination padlock I use only once a year at most, but I have remembered the combination for many years with an image of a cartoonish **ma** waving a frying pan and chasing **Nero** who is holding a **match** and rushing off to set fire to Rome (3-24-36). To remember my dentist appointment on the 26th at three o'clock, I imagine him smiling in an evil way to show a big **notch** between his front teeth while he works on a cartoonish **ma**. If I see an ad for a new restaurant I would like to try at 6541 Pine Street, I would imagine a **cello** player (65) entertaining a large **rat** (41) sitting in a pine tree.

Researchers have found that the major system can improve college students' memory for numbers provided they have access to the code words and are not rushed. Gary Patton and his collaborators gave students a short training session on the major system and then asked them to remember twenty two-digit numbers. Some students were given code words for the digit pairs, and others were asked to invent their own. Only those who were supplied with code words showed better performance than a control group that was given no memory aids at all. This surprised the researchers because it is usually better to create your own mnemonics rather than to use someone else's, but other studies have confirmed this finding with the major system. The lesson here is that a person who plans to use this approach should memorize a set of "canned" code words for the digits 0–99 rather than try to generate something on the spot.

With serious practice, the major system can help produce truly impressive number memory. Mnemonist and memory researcher Kenneth Higbee of Brigham Young University taught four students the major system and gave them forty hours of practice remembering numbers. Afterward, three of the four students were able to remember a fifty-digit number correctly after a three-minute exposure to it. The fourth student's best performance was forty-two digits out of fifty. Francis Bellezza, a researcher at Ohio University and also a mnemonist, taught a student the major system and worked with her as she practiced using it on long strings of digits presented one pair at a time on a computer screen. After about 100 hours of practice spread over one year, she could remember eighty-digit numbers with ninety-nine percent accuracy.

These efforts show what's possible after extensive practice, but real-world applications of the major system don't require anything like this level of training and commitment. After all, when would you ever want to remember an eighty-digit number? For the kinds of numbers we encounter in daily life—addresses, phone numbers, ID numbers, credit card numbers, prices, measurements, product numbers, dates, and times—a basic mastery of the major system is all that is necessary. You will find suggestions for getting up to speed on it in the Memory Lab section.

Variations

Memory competitors have modified the major system for use in memory contests. These innovations have been described as an "arms race" among competitors, a search for ways to encode memory information ever more quickly and efficiently. Ben Pridmore, a top British mnemonist, remembers numbers and dates with an expanded major system that includes separate codes for digits up to 1,000. Its advantage is that a long number can be memorized as a sequence of three-digit chunks rather than two-digit chunks as with the major system. This gives Pridmore fewer images to juggle when he tries to retain a long number. Of course, the downside is that his system requires massive practice to use effectively. Pridmore has employed it to give impressive performances, such as at the 2008 World Memory Championship, where he memorized 1,800 digits in one hour.

Dominic O'Brien, an eight-time world champion, developed a variant of the major system based on representing numbers with people—he associates a different person with numbers from 00 to 99. Each person is also associated with a characteristic action, so 13 is represented by Al Capone carrying a bottle of liquor, and 15 is Albert Einstein writing on a blackboard. The clever feature of this system is that it can encode a four-digit number with only one image. Say O'Brien wants to remember 1315. He imagines Al Capone (13) writing on a blackboard (15). By combining the person from the first two digits with the action from the second two, he can retain a long number with half as many images as the major system requires. Variations like O'Brien's and Pridmore's make sense for determined memory competitors who can justify the Olympian effort required to master and use them proficiently. But for a recreational mnemonist, these are systems to admire from a distance.

Chao Lu's System

The approach Chao Lu took to memorize 61,890 digits was similar to the major system. He tackled *pi* by working on groups of ten digits at a time, dividing each group into two-digit chunks. He then encoded each chunk as a concrete word using a set of codes he had established for the digits 00–99. He wove the code words for each ten digits into a vivid story. Here's the one he used for the first ten decimal places of *pi*: "a piece of a **rose** (14) was bitten off by a **parrot** (15) and delivered to **Lei Fang** (a famous Chinese soldier—92) at a **cow house** (65), who was smoking a **cigarette** (35)." Each story connected in some way to stories before and after it, creating long chains of narratives. Although the system was simple in principle, managing the massive number of stories required an enormous amount of memory rehearsal.

Chao Lu's strategy provided him with two essential aids for remembering numbers. The first turned a number into the kind of object the memory system can easily retain—one that is concrete, visual, and meaningful. His 00–99 code words did that. The next requirement was to bind the codes together so he could retrieve them from memory in the proper order, and that was the function of the stories he created. This two-pronged approach—one focused on encoding individual memory items and the other focused on organizing them—is common to other powerful memory devices, most notably the memory palaces that we'll talk about in Chapter 14.

A Final Thought

The numbers we encounter in life vary in importance, and some of them certainly should be recorded securely rather than trusted to memory. However, there are many others where a mnemonic strategy can be viable. It's true your pride will suffer if you botch it and have to backtrack to retrieve the number, but it is also true that this very possibility will motivate you to really work at it, and in the process increase your mnemonic skill. And remember that along the way you will be exercising your high-level mental abilities, relying on your own mental resources rather than external devices. These are the very cognitive processes most closely associated with intelligence and applicable to all manner of mental challenge.

The best way to get started remembering numbers is to practice the technique of finding a pattern. When the number is not too long, and when you will use it in the near future, this strategy can be all you need to retain it. The acrostic and number-shape approaches are useful in special circumstances. To progress further, a serious practitioner of the memory arts should consider taking on the major system. It is no walk in the park, to be sure, but it is quite doable at a level appropriate for a recreational mnemonist. You may find, as I have, that it is satisfying to master such a powerful system, and it puts you in the company of a long succession of mnemonists going back centuries.

In the Memory Lab:
How to Master the Major System

In this installment, we tackle learning the 110 code words that are essential for using the major system. The first step is to master the sounds associated with each digit as given earlier in the chapter. A memory cue for them is the sentence **Satan may relish coffee pie,** which decodes to 0123456789. A helper image is depicted below. Once the codes are secure in memory, you are ready to start on the 110 words. The table that appeared earlier (on page 149) gives the set of code words I use. If you don't like a word or find it hard to remember, think of a better one that decodes to the same number. Online resources are available to suggest code words for specific numbers— try searching for "major system word generator."

The best way to learn a list this long is in blocks. Start with the

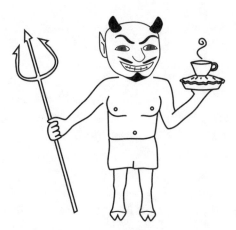

"Satan may relish coffee pie" is a mnemonic for remembering major system codes for the digits 0123456789.

first ten, and when you can recite them easily, go to the next ten. Each time you finish a block, run through the previous words to make sure you still have them. You'll find the cues provided by the consonants very helpful. If one of the words gives you trouble, substitute an alternate. What you want at this stage is to be able to reel off the 110 words in order.

Next, practice the codes in random order so that you'll be able to rapidly come up with the right word for any pair of digits. Flashcards are one way to get the job done. There are also online sites and cell phone apps to drill you on your code words. Find them by searching the Internet for "major system memory training." Space out your practice sessions and continue until the code words come to you easily. That is all there is to it. You will be ready to look for opportunities to put this effort to good use. And here is an added benefit: On those nights when you have trouble drifting off to sleep, just review the 110 code words: "zoo . . . tie . . . hen . . . ma . . . zzzzz . . . "

11

Remembering Skills

The barista behind the espresso machine looked at the code on the next cup in the queue—a medium-sized skinny vanilla latte—and moved into action. Put four pumps of sugar-free vanilla into the cup. Grind and tamp the coffee. Pull two shots of espresso and mix it with the vanilla. Measure the right amount of skim milk into a metal pitcher. And then the crucial step: Use the steam wand to aerate the milk and bring its temperature to 150 degrees. She completed the order by mixing the milk into the cup with just the right amount of foam on top. After she'd secured the lid, the latte was ready for the customer to pick up. The barista turned at once to the next cup. At this busy location, she sometimes pushes through 100 drinks an hour.

But this order was not finished. "Excuse me! Excuse me," the customer called out. "This latte is not hot enough." The barista may have been skeptical—her equipment is carefully maintained to get the temperature exactly right. In fact, the complaint could well be more about a coffee prima donna than the temperature of the drink. But if any of that passed through her consciousness, it didn't show, because her training kicked in. After establishing eye contact with the customer, she began to make things right. If she were a less experienced barista, she might have recalled the Starbucks acronym for dealing with unhappy customers—**LATTE:** Listen, Acknowledge, Take action, Thank the customer, and Explain what might have caused the problem. But she didn't need acronyms: She was a seasoned hand who knew how to respond to a customer problem, and she carried it out smoothly.

The barista's job is all about skill, not only the motor skills needed to operate the equipment, but also the cognitive and people skills she needs to interact with customers in a way that will keep them coming back for more. The barista, like all of us, possesses a broad range of skills that go far beyond her job, a skill collection that defines who she is as a person. Skills give us efficient, predictable ways to achieve our goals. They are at work when we prepare meals, drive cars, use computers, and play sports. They are at the core of the surgeon's technique, the stockbroker's advice, and the politician's deal making. As we saw in Chapter 1, skills rely on a specialized form of memory that is distinct from our memory for facts and personal experiences. You see evidence for this when you ask skilled people how they do what they do; they often cannot come up with a satisfactory explanation—their skill is something they can't put into words.

How Skills Are Acquired

The barista learned to make lattes by watching a trainer demonstrate the technique, an experience that left behind a memory of how to make one. This is how most skills start out: through the acquisition of basic knowledge that is retained as an explicit memory. The long-term memory systems described in Chapter 1, most of which are involved in learning a skill, are shown again below. The barista retained the trainer's demonstration as an episodic memory. She also knew a number of facts about lattes—the different varieties, the different sizes, her favorites—which she had picked up here and there before she took the barista job. She relied on this explicit knowledge at first. In fact, if we were to watch her closely as she prepared her first latte, we might have seen her lips moving ever so slightly as she mentally talked herself through the process by recalling what her trainer showed her. These were slow, inefficient productions, and they required

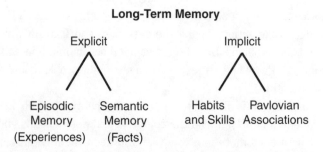

Long-Term Memory

Explicit

Episodic
Memory
(Experiences)

Semantic
Memory
(Facts)

Implicit

Habits
and Skills

Pavlovian
Associations

that she stay focused by devoting her cognitive resources exclusively to each step.

As our barista served up more lattes, we would see rapid improvement. Each time she successfully completed the required sequence, the behavior pattern was strengthened as a skill memory. This is a system specialized for carrying out efficient movements to achieve a specific goal. Unlike the explicit memory system, skill memory is established gradually, improving with each success, as illustrated in the graph below. We would see this as a series of small enhancements, like using the steam wand more deftly or pulling espresso shots more smoothly. She will also improve in a less obvious way by learning to pay attention to the things that matter—what to watch as she aerates the milk to get the right amount of foam and how to judge the quality of a shot as she pulls it. These perceptual skills are every bit as important as the motor skills involved in operating the machine. With each advance, the skill becomes better established in her implicit memory system and less dependent on her explicit, conscious knowledge. She moves from "knowing that" (explicit knowledge) to "knowing how" (skill).

More practice will lead to easier and smoother operations until they are so secure she can exchange pleasantries with a customer as she works or even allow her thoughts to drift to topics far removed from her espresso machine. These are distractions she wouldn't have been able to manage previously without spoiling a drink. Psychologists describe the behavior as automatic because it requires little conscious control.

The fact that automatic skills are almost effortless leads to huge benefits when the skill is embedded in a complex process. A pianist whose finger movements for a well-practiced piece have become largely automatic is able to apply her cognitive resources to the work's expressiveness, giving

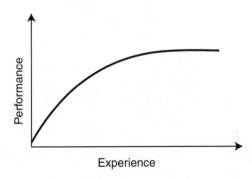

it gaiety, excitement, or surprise. A less practiced performer must reserve conscious attention to handle fingering details. The expert surgeon who has practiced specialized procedures to the point where they are automatic frees up his high-level mental abilities to handle unexpected problems and to plan the next steps.

Some skills are more about mental operations than physical movements—handling an unhappy customer, programming a computer, controlling air traffic, or memorizing the order of a deck of playing cards. Interestingly, their development is similar to more physical skills like playing a piano or using a scalpel. At first these skills are dependent on explicit knowledge consciously remembered and put to use, step by step. The new chess player needs to recall the way pawns and rooks, kings and queens move and then sort through the options available for each. But with practice, the basics of play become automatic and players become able to use their cognitive resources for more strategic and complex aspects of the game.

Mnemonic skills develop in the same way. Say you want to become better at remembering names by using the strategy from Chapter 7 cued by the acrostic "Friendly Llamas Seek People"—**F**ind a feature, **L**isten to the name, **S**ay it back, and **P**ractice. Initially, it will take effort to hold the four steps in mind, and you may even need the helper image repeated below. At this stage you are relying on explicit memory to carry out the strategy. But as with the barista at the espresso machine, each success strengthens

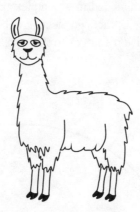

The Friendly Llama, a helper image used to recall an acrostic relevant for learning a name.

the process as a skill memory, and the routine becomes easier to follow. More practice also leads to refinements as you learn how to spot people's distinguishing features, what to do with difficult names, how to mentally practice new names, how to work names into conversations. You become less and less dependent on explicit memories for guidance, and you find it takes less attention and mental effort to carry out the steps. Eventually you won't need the Friendly Llama at all because your implicit memory system will be directing the action. The key steps now occur almost effortlessly, making the mnemonic superfluous.

Getting from "Good Enough" to "Good"

Most skills will get to a point where your performance no longer improves with practice. You may discover your tennis skill is stuck at an intermediate level no matter how often you play. Your cooking may not be soaring to culinary heights, even though you put dinner on the table every night. What's happened is that your practice is maintaining the status quo: Your skills aren't getting sharper, but they're not diminishing either.

What separates you from others who continue to improve? Motivation certainly plays a part. It could well be that you are at peace with your performance and have no serious interest in improving. Many skills are like that. Whether it's playing softball, making home repairs, or managing investments, many of us are satisfied with a skill level far short of real expertise.

But what about skills you would like to improve? Motivation alone isn't enough to bring this about. You've always wanted to be a better cook, but it just isn't happening. And then there's your tennis game. The development of expertise requires more than just wanting it. In fact, studies of high achievers reveal that they make focused efforts to hone their skills. Psychologist Anders Ericsson, a leader in this research, has studied top performers in areas as diverse as chess, music, medicine, bridge, computer programming, sports, and memory skill. These are individuals whose performance curves have risen way above the level of "good enough" as shown on the graph on the next page. Ericsson and his colleagues discovered common elements in the ways elite achievers practiced. For them practice is a serious endeavor. They work to get as much gain as possible from each session; they reflect on what was successful, and they figure out how to do

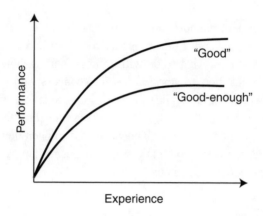

better. Ericsson called this "deliberate practice," and it applies to a Sunday golfer as much as to an Olympic hopeful. He found three features of deliberate practice that work together to keep skill development moving forward, putting it on a trajectory to become "good."

1. Target Specific Improvements

The best way to improve skills is to focus on specifics. The tennis player may work on her serve, the cook on his sautéing technique. The barista, having mastered the fundamentals, might decide to upgrade her technique for steaming milk so that she can consistently produce the finely aerated, creamy foam of top-quality lattes. By singling out foam for improvement, she leaves other parts of the skill as they are, largely automatic steps she performs easily. Focusing on the foam process changes it from being automatic to being consciously controlled. She can now apply her attention, working memory, and reasoning abilities to improve it. There can be no chatting with customers at this stage because she will need her cognitive resources to work out the fine points of making better foam. It is no surprise that Ericsson and his colleagues have found that improvement is demanding mental work.

An important part of deliberate practice is problem solving. The barista must figure out how to get the steam wand to produce small rather than large bubbles in the milk and then learn how to stir them into the creamy texture she wants. It will take repeated tries, but if she stays focused, it is within her grasp, and with even more practice the new routine will become largely automatic. At this point she can talk to customers and still produce high-quality foam.

2. Value Feedback

Unless the barista can determine the quality of the foam she is producing, she can't improve—feedback is essential for deliberate practice to work. In her case, a more experienced coworker could serve as a coach to provide feedback and suggest practice goals. In fact, this is the ideal situation for skill development. In the world of elite performers, coaches and trainers are highly prized for just these reasons. If the barista can find such a person, she will be able to improve her skills quickly.

When finding a coach isn't practical, you must look for another way to solve the feedback problem. Say you're a mnemonist who wants to improve your memory for names. What feedback will be most useful? And how can you get that feedback? Simply knowing how many names you remembered from an event isn't specific enough to help you improve your technique. You would do better to find a time soon after the event to reflect, a time when you can still recall how well you performed on each of the four Friendly Llama steps. You may make notes on your observations while your memory is fresh and then work out practice goals for your next opportunity. Each skill presents its own challenge. Finding a practical way to get feedback must be a priority for anyone interested in improving because without it, practice only reinforces errors and inefficiencies.

3. Get Lots of Practice

There is one more essential ingredient in deliberate practice: it has to be repeated over and over. How much practice? That depends on the complexity of the skill and the aspirations of the performer. In competitive fields like music, chess, surgery, or science, elite achievers typically invest ten years of serious work to become top performers.

That kind of commitment is out of reach for a recreational golfer, musician, or mnemonist. The amount of practice they can manage is not only compromised by other life interests, but it also can be undermined by the logistics of finding practice opportunities. How they juggle priorities, find opportunities, and marshal self-discipline will determine where they wind up on the continuum between "good enough" and "good."

Mental Rehearsal

Not all practice has to involve activities in the outside world. It can also take place in the mind. Top athletes use mental rehearsal as part of their practice for competitive events. Here is a successful Olympian springboard diver talking about his preparation:

> I did my dives in my head all the time. At night, before going to sleep, I always did my dives. Ten dives. I started with a front dive, the first one I had to do at the Olympics, and I did everything as if I was actually there. I saw myself on the board with the same bathing suit. Everything was the same. . . . If the dive was wrong, I went back and started over again. It takes a good hour to do perfect imagery of all my dives, but it was better than a workout.

Mental imagery has become a fixture in Olympic training circles. At the 2014 Sochi Winter Games, the United States brought nine sports psychologists to assist athletes in preparing for their events, and using imagery to improve skills was a major focus. Earlier studies of Olympic contenders have shown that the most successful competitors reported using more imagery than the less successful ones.

The idea that you can improve a skill by mentally practicing it is a well-researched principle in psychology. It is supported not only for sports but also for performing surgery, playing music, executing dance routines, landing airplanes, carrying out laboratory tasks, and recovering from strokes.

If you decide to give mental practice a try, it's best to wait until you've mastered the basics of the skill with hands-on practice and you're familiar with environments where it will be used. This is important because mental rehearsal works best when your imagined performance closely mimics the actual physical sensations of performing the skill—and you will need experience to be able to construct this imagery. The correspondence between real and imaginary should be as close as you can manage, starting with how the setting will look to you as you perform the skill, even what you will be wearing. The sensations of physical movements are an important part of mental rehearsal. The pianist should be able to feel her fingers working the keys; a softball pitcher should feel the windup before the mental throw; and a mnemonist should feel the pressure of a handshake during the imagined introduction. Even the emotions that accompany the skill—being nervous or feeling excited—will make the imagery more realistic and thus more effective.

Suppose you want to improve your ability to remember names of people you meet at a party or a business conference. You could picture yourself carrying out the Friendly Llama strategy successfully and retaining the names of imaginary people you will meet at a forthcoming event. Ideally, you will have been to the actual room where the introductions will take place so you can visualize it in your mind, but if not, you will need to picture a similar setting. You will see yourself there in the clothes you'll be wearing, and you will imagine behaving as you hope to behave at the real event. I recommend that you prepare a written script to guide the imagery, especially at first. Here is an example:

> *I am coming into the room for the meeting . . . I'm wearing my blue sports coat and gray trousers . . . no tie today . . . I am carrying my tablet. . . . I see the setup, the chairs, the table, the screen, the coffee urn. . . . I recall my retention intention for today . . . I seriously want to learn as many new names as I can. . . . I am looking forward to it and feeling pumped about my prospects. . . . I start noticing people I don't know . . . I check them out. . . . I wonder who they are and what they are like . . . I look for distinguishing features . . . I nod to a woman I know . . . she is standing with a man I want to meet . . . I have picked out a feature I can use to remember this guy—it's his abundant head of hair—and note it as I go over . . . I feel my legs moving as I go over to where she is . . . we say hello . . . as she begins to introduce me to the new person, I make eye contact . . . I give him my full attention . . . I feel my arm extend . . . I experience the handshake . . . I keep my full attention on him as he says his name . . . I hear him say "Jay" . . . I repeat it . . . "Glad to meet you, Jay" . . . I note his distinguishing feature again . . . we talk . . . I mentally repeat his name to myself . . . I excuse myself to say hello to someone else . . . I repeat "Nice meeting you, Jay" as I leave. . . .*

Scripts can be about more than just the skill; they can also create motivation, as this one does, and they can prepare you to cope with difficulties you might encounter. For example, you could get overwhelmed when you're being introduced to a lot of people, one after the other. You may know from experience that once that sinking feeling hits, you tend to give up trying to retain the names. Instead of giving up, prepare yourself for this situation by adding a section to the script in which you imagine that it happens and you deal with it. You might see yourself becoming overwhelmed, recognize what is happening, and respond by turning your attention inward, taking a breath, refocusing, and then going back to the Friendly Llama strategy. By rehearsing a coping response in advance, you increase the chances you can pull it off at the real event.

You can work from a written script or you can read it into a recording device and play it back to yourself. In either case, the goal is to create the images it describes. As you experiment with mental rehearsal, keep in mind that it is itself a skill and takes practice to master. Its two key requirements are making the imagery as vivid as you can and controlling it so that you can accurately portray the skill you are practicing.

You can use this rehearsal technique either to develop a skill or to prepare for a specific occasion. When you use it for development, it will be most effective in conjunction with actual practice. When you use it to tune up a skill for an upcoming event, the method will work best if you carry it out close to the time when you will need the skill.

The Leaky Bucket Problem

Just because you master a skill doesn't mean you will always perform it well. Suppose you successfully complete a training course in cardiopulmonary resuscitation (CPR). Will you be able to carry it out successfully if you encounter an emergency in six months? In a year? There will almost certainly be some drop in performance, but how much? That was the question British researcher Ian Glendon and his colleagues asked in a study of shop-floor and office workers who took a CPR course from professional instructors. Those who performed well were recruited to come back for a retest after different periods of time. When they arrived for the test, they were taken to a room where they found a "casualty," a manikin instrumented to record details of the CPR effort. This allowed experts to judge whether each participant would have maintained a real person's vital functions well enough to allow survival. The graph on the facing page shows how skill levels lapsed in a major way over the one-year period. After twelve and a half months, only fourteen percent of the CPR attempts would have been adequate to save the victim.

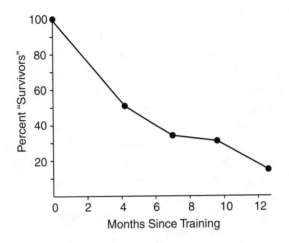

CPR competency in the months following CPR training.

This is the leaky bucket problem—a loss of competence over time when you don't practice a skill. Just how much loss depends on the skill. You are not likely to forget how to swim or ride a bike, even if you don't practice. The simple structure of repetitive movements guided by environmental cues makes these activities resistant to decay. But when a skill is replete with multiple steps and time pressures, it can degrade quickly. This is what happened in the CPR study, because CPR requires that a sequence of actions be performed precisely at a specified rate with little feedback available to signal its being done correctly. Over time there is slippage—steps can drop out, the compressions can become too shallow, the tempo can become too rushed. Regular practice is the only remedy. The Red Cross recommends a CPR refresher every three months, and the graph shows this is none too soon.

With more complex skills, practice must be even more frequent or performance will suffer. The great pianist Ignacy Paderewski famously observed, "If I miss one day's practice, I notice it. If I miss two days' practice, the critics notice it. If I miss three days' practice, the public notices it." Other demanding skills are similar in their practice requirements. A typical F-15 pilot must fly thirteen practice sorties a month to maintain adequate proficiency for real missions. And when it comes to the Olympics, hopefuls organize their lives around practice, both real and imaginary.

A Final Thought

Many people who take my memory classes hope to learn techniques that will instantly give them a better memory. Of course, it doesn't work that way, no more than learning how a latte is made will instantly make you a competent barista. In any complex skill, expert performance comes from an interplay between the explicit and implicit memory systems, an interplay that requires practice. This insight is especially important for anyone who aspires to be a practitioner of the memory arts. Because it's a skill based on techniques that can be described easily, it's seductive to believe that knowledge of the techniques is all you need. But explicit knowledge is only a starting point. An appropriate amount of deliberate practice must take place because practical utility won't come until the techniques become established as smoothly flowing procedures in the implicit memory system.

In the Memory Lab:
The Link Method

This installment of the Memory Lab introduces a useful way to remember a series of memory items in a specific order. We look at an example of the method here, and then in Chapter 13 we'll examine it more thoroughly.

The Link Method is especially useful when you want to move easily from one item in a series to the next. For example, imagine you're working your way through a mental grocery list. You've just picked up the butter, and now you need the next item on the list. The Link Method will help bring it to mind.

Here we construct a memory aid for recalling the three components of deliberate practice in order. To add a practical context, suppose I'm preparing to deliver a lecture on this material, and I don't want to rely on notes. The Link Method allows me to move through the topics in order without external memory aids. Although the application here involves only three topics, the process could be extended to link as many topics as I wished.

The three components of deliberate practice are (1) target specific aspects of the skill, (2) get feedback on performance, and (3) practice. To apply the Link Method, I create associations between the pairs of components in the order I want to recall them.

To improve skills →
      Target specifics →
            Get feedback →
                  Practice

Every arrow will become a visual image linking the items on either side of it. The diagram shows I need three visual images to create the three links.

First Link: To Improve Skills → Target Specifics

I used a juggler to suggest skills and a bull's-eye to represent targeting specifics, as shown below. Combining them by showing bull's-eye targets being juggled gave the association I was looking for. During the lecture, when I get to improving skills, I mentally look for an association to that topic, and I recall the juggler image. The bull's-eyes will help me remember the first component of deliberate practice: targeting specifics of the skill.

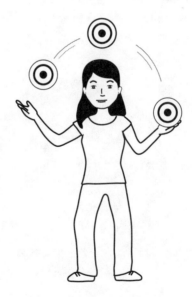

The first of three images to link together the steps involved in deliberate practice. Here skill learning (the juggler) is associated with targeting a specific skill component (the targets).

Second Link: Target Specifics → Get Feedback

An interesting feature of the Link Method is that each association is independent of the others. So, to create the second link, I put the juggler aside and looked for something to connect "targeting specifics" and "feedback." Because "feedback" is abstract and not easily represented as a visual image, I looked for a substitute word that could suggest "feedback." I chose "food" and then imagined a target with "food" in the center, as depicted below. This will be enough to get me to recall "feedback." During the lecture, as I finish talking about targeting specifics, I mentally look for an association with "targeting," recall this image, and know the next topic is "feedback."

Third Link: Get Feedback → Practice

When I'm ready to make the third point, I will search for an association with feedback and recall the third link, shown on the facing page. It displays a hapless musician being pelted with hostile feedback as a disappointed audience hurls tomatoes. He obviously needs more practice, an implication that will cue the last topic. As you look at these images, keep in mind that effective memory cues are idiosyncratic.

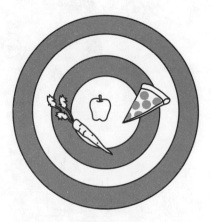

The next visual image used in the link method. The second step of deliberate practice, getting feedback, is connected with the previous step, targeting a specific skill component.

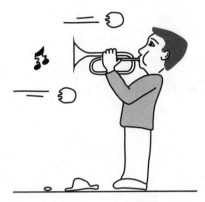

The final link for remembering the three steps of deliberate practice. It associates feedback with more practice.

These images work for me, but if you were delivering the lecture and using the Link Method, your images would likely be different.

Once I have the links, I run through them in my mind several times before the lecture to make sure they will come easily to me as I move from topic to topic. If I choose the link images well, I'll be comfortable speaking without notes, and the lecture will follow the path I intend for it.

12

Remembering Life

James McGaugh is a leading authority on memory. As a top researcher, he has published scores of scientific papers and has been lauded for his major insights about the memory system. It was because of his prominence that Jill Price emailed him on June 8, 2000:

> I am thirty-four years old and since I was eleven I have had this unbelievable ability to recall my past, but not just recollections. My first memories are of being a toddler in a crib (circa 1967) however I can take a date between 1974 and today, and tell you what day it falls on, what I was doing that day, and if anything of great importance . . . occurred that day I can describe that to you as well. I do not look at calendars beforehand and I do not read twenty-four years of my journals either. Whenever I see a date flash on the television (or anywhere else for that matter) I automatically go back to that day and remember where I was, what I was doing, what day it fell on and on and on and on and on. It is non-stop, uncontrollable and totally exhausting.

Ms. Price hoped that McGaugh, Larry Cahill, and their colleagues at the University of California, Irvine, could help her gain some control of her memories so that they were not so draining of her energy. McGaugh agreed to a meeting, but he was deeply skeptical that her memory could be that remarkable. Researchers call this form of remembering "autobiographical memory," and everything that was known about it then suggested that what she claimed was impossible.

As McGaugh's team put Price through an extensive series of memory tests, it became clear that she indeed had phenomenal autobiographical memory. Her old journals allowed the researchers to test her recollections against what she had written years earlier. Her memories invariably checked out. In one surprise test, they asked her to write down the date that Easter fell on each year between 1980 and 2003. Not only did she give the dates, but she also volunteered what she had been doing on each day. For example, she reported that on Easter Sunday, March 30, 1986, her parents were in Palm Springs and three friends were staying with her at their house. In 1989, Easter was on March 26, and she remembered spending it with a friend. The journal entries matched her memories.

Interestingly, the tests showed that Price's memory for other types of information—numbers, words, pictures, and diagrams—was undistinguished. She reported that she had trouble remembering school material. But for life events that she found interesting or personally relevant, her memory was jaw-dropping.

McGaugh and Cahill studied Price's memory over several years and documented capabilities never previously suspected by researchers. Price patiently assisted their efforts, and over time she began to make peace with her extraordinary memory, eventually writing a book, *The Woman Who Can't Forget,* about the role it had played in her life.

Word about McGaugh's work spread, and other people with similar abilities were discovered. Unlike Price, they valued their uncommon proficiency. But like Price, they could recall daily experiences for calendar dates picked at random, and their memories checked out, just as hers did. McGaugh and his team carefully studied many of them with interviews, memory tests, and even brain scans. They named this rare ability "highly superior autobiographical memory" (HSAM). I will come back to what they learned about it, but first consider how the rest of us remember our past. It's totally different, and it will provide a context to appreciate these special people and see what they have to teach us if we want to remember our own lives better.

What We Remember

Those of us without Jill Price's abilities will forget most of what happens to us in life. It's true that each day adds new memories—the conversation at breakfast, the search for a parking space, the meeting with a colleague, the lunch at the deli. These events will usually be recallable for days, weeks, or even longer when a good memory cue is available—if you go back to that deli next month, you may still be able to recall details of what you and a friend talked about. Nonetheless, most of this information is doomed to be forgotten. But not all of it. What is it about the memories we retain?

Gillian Cohen and Dorothy Faulkner, two British researchers, attempted to find out by asking 154 people between twenty and eighty-seven years of age to identify their most vivid memories and to write a few words about each. The bar chart below shows the top nine themes in the memories people recalled. Taken together they account for over eighty percent of all memories reported. What is it about these events that allowed them to be remembered while so many others were lost to time? Cohen and Faulkner believe that each one was (1) personally important, or (2) unusual, or (3) emotionally significant, or some combination of these qualities.

The memory advantage of novel events deserves special note. The ease with which we retain the odd, the rare, the unusual, and the unexpected is shown by the fact that seventy-three percent of memories found in that study involved situations that are not routine—a first love, a trip abroad, an illness. The memorability of such distinctive experiences is dramatically illustrated in a study by David Pillemer and his colleagues at Wellesley College. They tracked down graduates who had been out of school for twenty-two years and asked them what they remembered from their first year of college. As the graph on the facing page shows, most of these memo-

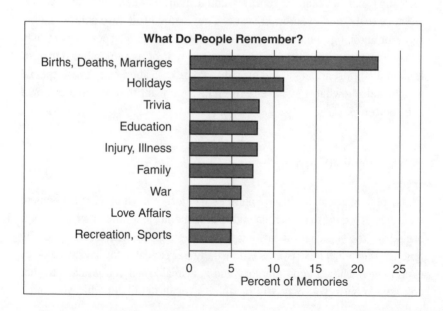

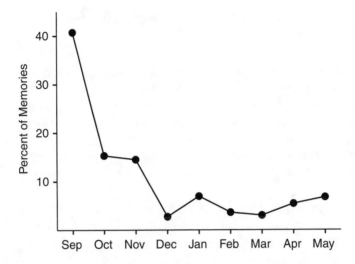

First-year college memories after twenty-two years.

ries came from one month—the month they arrived. This was when they encountered one fresh experience after another as they met roommates, talked with advisors, found their way around campus, and attended classes. These first-time experiences left lasting impressions. Later experiences, on the other hand, were "same old, same old," not distinctive enough to register well in memory.

Feelings are the other powerful memory enhancer. This was evident in the Wellesley study, where the great majority of remembrances were linked to emotion. You'll find the same is true of your own long-lasting memories. If you go back to your experience of college or high school and pay attention to the first memories that come to mind, they will most certainly have an emotional component that helped make them memorable—those first high school dances, accomplishments with the photo club, camaraderie at a football game.

Emotion has a special relationship to memory because of its ability to strengthen memories as they are created. The neurochemicals that accompany emotion affect the brain areas where memories are formed, and the result is a vivid, durable representation of the event. A notable example is a "flashbulb memory," an emotional experience preserved in compelling detail and capable of lasting a lifetime. Following is an elderly Danish man's memory of the invasion of Denmark on April 9, 1940, when he was thirteen years old.

> I was woken up by a thundering noise, never heard anything like it. Opened the skylight in the attic and looked towards the south. Over the woods nearby, squadrons of big grey planes are coming, three at a time, right above the tree-tops. One can see the pilots in their cockpits, and the sides of the planes are wavy sheet metal with big black and white crosses on them. I run downstairs to my family—consisting of my mother and grandmother. My mother is furious. The radio has announced that we are occupied by the Germans.

This memory had a lot going for it. Not only was the event important and unusual, but it also evoked strong emotions. In fact, it was probably the emotional content that's responsible for its crystal clarity and many details, the signature characteristics of flashbulb memories. Danish psychologists Dorthe Berntsen and Dorthe Thomsen used a variety of methods to check the accuracy of flashbulb memories recalled by elderly Danes who had lived through the invasion. Most checked out as substantially correct despite a retention period of more than sixty years.

A more recent event that produced flashbulb memories for many was the September 11, 2001, attack on the World Trade Center in New York. If you were old enough at the time, you probably have a clear memory of hearing about it. Is that memory coming back right now? Can you say where you were and what you were doing? How you learned about the attack? What you did next? If you can answer these questions, you have a flashbulb memory, and you are not alone. Not only do Americans who were at least adolescents at the time overwhelmingly remember it well, so also do residents of Britain, Belgium, Italy, Romania, Japan, and other countries. This was a flashbulb event worldwide.

In the Middle Ages, emotion was intentionally deployed for mnemonic purposes in powerful ways, creating flashbulb memories in the process. Here is historian Morris Bishop describing those times:

> Another curious aspect of medieval justice was the method of impressing dates and decisions on witnesses' memories, since written records were scanty or inaccessible. Boys who served as witnesses were solemnly cuffed or flogged to vivify their memory until old age. Coultron records that "Roger de Montgomery had thrown into the water his son Robert of Bellême, clad in a

fur coat, ... in testimony and in memorial that the [property] of the abbot and his monks extended as far as that point."

By associating an emotional experience with a crucial fact, the medieval judge ensured that the location of the abbot's property line would be safe with young Robert for a long time as a flashbulb memory. Similarly, those who served as witnesses to marriages would sometimes follow the ceremony by hitting one another to make sure they remembered the union, a serious responsibility in a time with no formal record keeping.

Emotional memories are usually relatively accurate, but not always. In fact, sometimes they contain vivid and compelling errors. Consider flashbulb memories for September 11, 2001. Several days after the attack Lia Kvavilashvili and her colleagues at the University of Hertfordshire asked a large sample of people to describe how they had heard about it. They contacted the same people two years later and asked them to remember the event again. About ten percent of their participants showed major distortions in what they remembered. For example, a day after the event, one woman recalled that she had heard about the attack when she went to pick up her granddaughter at a playground. Two years later, she remembered hearing about it from a clerk in a dry cleaning establishment. She recalled both memories vividly. Instances like this show a risk associated with emotional memories. Because they seem so real, we accept them uncritically. But an impressive body of research shows that they regularly contain errors. The lesson for us as students of memory is to keep in mind that vivid memories are not guaranteed to be accurate. Any memory, even a flashbulb experience, can be in error.

The Bump

Suppose you write down the first fifty memories of your life you can think of. It will turn out that quite a few of them will be from the last year or so, but put those aside and look only at the older memories. What periods of your life did they come from? If you are over fifty, you'll find a disproportionate number of memories from the time when you were fifteen to thirty years old. This "bump" is illustrated in the graph on page 176, derived from studies of people in their seventies who were given a series of cue words

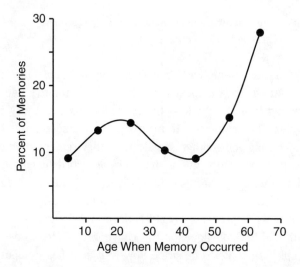

An autobiographical bump occurs between the ages of fifteen and thirty when people over fifty recall memories from their lives.

like *cat, flower,* and *ticket* and asked to recall a memory for each word. When scientists plotted the ages those events occurred, they discovered "the bump." This has turned out to be a surprisingly robust finding. It not only holds for memories spontaneously recalled and memories triggered by cue words, but also for memories cued by odors or recalled in life stories.

The bump is probably due to a combination of factors. It seems no coincidence that it occurs in the years when the cognitive system is at peak efficiency, when people score their highest on memory tests and when their reaction times are the quickest. It is also a crucial time for social development. During these years we navigate adolescence and find our adult identity. Major chapters in our life story are written as we take on college, careers, marriage, and children. These many experiences will often have all the features associated with strong memories—personal importance, novelty, and emotional content. It is indeed a special time of life, and the bump reflects it.

What about Earlier Memories?

Just as the bump represents our best remembered years, the period before it qualifies as the worst. When adults are asked to recall early memories, they seldom remember experiences before about the age of three. Freud called this dearth "childhood amnesia." It's not that children younger than three don't remember things; it's that their memories don't last. Even by the time a child is six, memory for the early years has largely faded. Part of the reason is brain development. Key memory structures are too immature in very young children for them to hold on to their experiences for very long. There are also social factors at work. Children have to learn how to put the bits and pieces of their remembered experiences together to form coherent stories of what happened. Interactions with their parents and other adults gradually teach this skill. As they get better at expressing their existing memories, the children's retention of new information also improves. By the time they are eight or nine, both nature and nurture have brought their memory systems to a point where their new memories are as robust as those formed by adults.

The Life Story

Another milestone in memory development occurs as people move into their teenage years and begin to organize their memories into a life story. This is a time when adolescents face a daunting agenda: establish gender identity, deal with tricky peer relationships, sort out educational options, and work through changing family dynamics. These challenges prompt interest in their own stories, an interest seen in the tendency of many teens to keep a diary—about a third of the college students I teach say they did so during these years. The life stories they are beginning to formulate will continue to evolve throughout their lives, and as this happens, memories will link together to capture different aspects of their experiences. An after-school job in high school will leave behind more than a bunch of isolated memories. Instead, the memories will form a story about this activity during those years, a narrative involving people, events, emotions, and responsibilities, all with special meaning for the person involved. Researchers call collections of memories like this a "chapter" in the life story. Memories from other aspects of a person's life will form other chapters—the years in the college dorm, a serious romantic relationship, a parent's illness. Each chapter pulls together memories of related events into a narrative structure that gives context and meaning. As the years pass, the life story will be expanded, updated, edited, revised, and reinterpreted. It serves as our per sonal perspective on the past, one that shapes how we see the present and how we look toward the future.

Because life stories organize autobiographical memories, they can play a role in retrieving them. Martin Conway, a prominent researcher, has theorized that such memories are organized as a hierarchy with three levels. At the highest level are collections of memories ordered chronologically according to a particular theme to form a chapter, such as "my years in the dorm." A second level consists of situations in the chapter where a group of memories took place. For example, "my freshman roommate, Jared," identifies a general situation with many dorm memories. At the lowest level in Conway's hierarchy are memories of specific episodes like "the time Jared screwed up my computer."

To see the system in action, suppose my wife asks if I remember the small garden she planted years ago when we lived in California. How will I locate that memory among the many thousands of experiences I've had? It may be that the cue she gave me, "small garden in California," will be enough to let me immediately retrieve the memory, but since this was long ago, directly retrieving it could well fail. If so, I might still be able to find the memory if I come at it from my life story as shown in the box below. I would begin by mentally going back to those California years, a chapter in my life story, and recalling a duplex we lived in at the time. This setting is associated with many memories, and it's where I would have experienced the garden. There I discover cues to bring the garden memory to mind—and to remember how much we enjoyed the taste of those tomatoes right off the vine. The life story, with its hierarchical organization, provides an alternate access to personal memories. It is slower and less efficient than a good cue

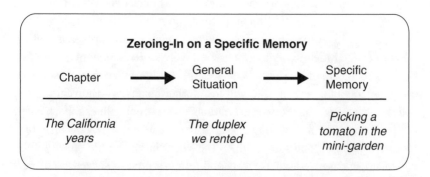

that takes us directly to the memory, but it can save the day when available cues are inadequate.

Highly Superior Autobiographical Memory (HSAM)

What about those people like Jill Price who have such amazing memories for autobiographical experiences? How do they do it? Can we learn anything from them that will help us better remember our own lives?

Although many questions remain, there have been enlightening discoveries about those with HSAM. Four scientific articles have now appeared about them as well as two books by HSAM individuals. In addition to Jill Price's story, Marilu Henner has written a self-help book titled *Total Memory Makeover.* Henner is an accomplished actress and author of other self-help books on health and diet. Her new book describes her HSAM and makes recommendations to readers about ways to improve their ability to remember their pasts. I'll come back to her suggestions later. One key finding about HSAM is enthrallment with the calendar. Those with HSAM can give the day of the week for any date as long as it's in the period of their lives where they have detailed memory, usually after about the age of eleven or twelve. They know when leap years occur, which months have identical calendar pages, and which years are identical for all months. Their memories are tied to specific dates, and this gives them a way to organize their memories so they can recall them easily and systematically. And with each rehearsal, the memories become stronger. Jill Price recalls that December 19, 1980, was the last day of school in tenth grade just before Christmas vacation. On December 19, 1981, she went shopping with Dean and Harry in Beverly Hills. She can continue remembering December 19ths right up to the present. It is striking how ordinary her memories for these dates are. These are not important events or especially noteworthy or charged with strong emotions; they are just daily happenings, the kind of things the rest of us easily forget. By tying the events to dates, she created specific cues that allow her to remember them, and she does this frequently. For example, as she blow-dries her hair each morning, she mentally flips back through the same day of the month in previous years to recall what happened. Marilu Henner and others with HSAM report similar practices.

Perhaps not surprisingly, a commonality among people with HSAM is a marked tendency toward obsessiveness—not enough to qualify as a psychological disorder but definitely more than the average person. They collect and carefully organize clothing, music CDs, mugs, hats, stuffed animals, and *TV Guide*s. The McGaugh team believes their need for order and their tendency toward obsessiveness may be linked to HSAM. It could explain their calendar fascination as a way to organize their memories, and it could motivate their habitual rehearsal of past years.

There is one other common element among these remarkable people: Those who have it value their special ability. None of the individuals studied, not even Jill Price, would give up their special memory if they could. One woman, Louise Owen, put it like this: "I think it makes me live my life with so much more intention and so much more joy. . . . I know that I am going to remember whatever happens today. What can I do to make today special? What can I do to make today stand out?"

Strengthening Autobiographical Memory

Is there anything we can learn from HSAM people to improve our autobiographical memory? Actually, any of us could adopt some of their practices: they are people who deeply value memories of the past; they enjoy the process of reminiscing, and they rehearse their memories on a regular basis. Although their calendar abilities seem out of reach, most of us can improve our ability to reminiscence, and we can choose to take more pleasure in reviewing our past.

Of course, not everybody needs to improve. Some people frequently recall events from their past and enjoy doing so. Deliberate autobiographical remembering is a part of who they are. Other people, though, are much less reflective and don't intentionally access their autobiographical memories unless there is a practical reason for it. In between these extremes are all manner of gradations. As a general rule, women engage in autobiographical remembering more than men. They typically recall past experiences more vividly and report them in more detail, giving special prominence to the thoughts and feelings involved in the event.

The suggestions here are for those not given to autobiographical reflection who would like to strengthen it. After all, memory of our lives is arguably our most important possession, the basis for our sense of self and the storehouse for life's lessons. It seems worthy of effort if it isn't getting the attention you think it deserves.

A word of caution: not all autobiographical remembering is healthy. When people ruminate about old hurts or lost opportunities, or when they reminisce to escape the present, or when they dwell on memories of people no longer present, they make themselves vulnerable to depression. Constructive reminiscing takes two forms. It's healthy to review your life and the path you've followed, to appreciate who you are and how you came to be that way. You may recall experiences that became turning points in your life and reminisce about them to discover what they meant for you, experiences like the one this student reported:

> In my sophomore year, I took an English literature course. I loved the course material, enjoyed writing papers, and felt pretty good about it until . . . I wrote an essay on my interpretation of a poem. I felt I had great insight into a special meaning within the verse. When the paper was returned, the teacher told me I didn't have any understanding of the material and she hoped I wasn't going to be an English major. I remember her pinched face and small, tight mouth as she said these things to me. I thought no way do I want to be like her. So I changed my major from English to Sociology.

Reminiscing also serves as a learning tool because it allows you to look at how you handled situations in the past. Consider the memory that basketball superstar Michael Jordan has about the time he failed to make the varsity basketball team when he was a sophomore:

> It was embarrassing, not making that team. They posted the roster and it was there for a long, long time without my name on it. I remember being really mad, too, because there was a guy who made it that really wasn't as good as me. . . . Whenever I was working out and got tired and figured I ought to stop, I'd close my eyes, and see that list in the locker room without my name on it, and that usually got me going again.

Most memories won't have as strong an impact as these. They will be a mix of experiences, some positive, some negative, some neutral. For most people, the overwhelming majority of autobiographical memories will be positive—studies typically find a ratio of positive to negative memories of more than two to one. It may be for this reason that constructive reminiscing promotes positive feelings and a sense of well-being. In fact, constructive reminiscing under the guidance of a psychotherapist is a recognized treatment for depression. With that background, here are suggestions for improving autobiographical memory.

Acquiring Strong Memories

A good first step is to put extra effort into acquiring rich autobiographical memories in the first place. When I was in Seattle not too long ago, I had an opportunity to have dinner with my sister, her partner, her two daughters, and one of their husbands. It is rare for all of us to be together. I wanted to remember the occasion well, so I adopted the three-step process Marilu Henner recommends for situations like this: Anticipate—Participate—Recollect. She learned it from her father who also valued memory. He engaged her entire family in carrying out the three steps for festive occasions like Christmas gatherings, beach parties, and birthdays. Henner has warm memories of these experiences, and to this day she follows her father's process.

In my case, I approached the anticipate phase by looking ahead to the event with positive expectations, making plans to remember what would take place. This gave me a sense of mission during the event that I think increased my enjoyment. The next step, participate, occurred at the dinner, where I made a conscious effort to fully experience what transpired so that I could form strong memories. As the evening passed, I found myself noting certain moments that seemed especially worth remembering. The final step took place back in Anchorage several days later when I chose a quiet place to travel back in time and relive the event. The result was a rich memory for that experience.

What to Reminisce About

You may find it useful to spend some time identifying aspects of your life story that would be interesting to reminisce about. These could be experiences that helped shape your personality and values, or added richness to your life, or taught important lessons, or simply are rewarding to revisit. Here are three suggestions for finding them.

Major Chapters in Your Life Story

Say you divided your life into its most important segments. What would they be? These are the chapters I am referring to here. A chapter can be whatever you want it to be, but for me, memories in a chapter have a common theme; they cover an extended time period like weeks, months, or years; and they have a distinct chronological order. Marilu Henner suggests identifying life-story chapters by imagining you are going to write an autobiography or produce a documentary about yourself. How would the story develop? The box below shows chapter possibilities based on her suggestions and other sources. In one study of middle-aged people, the average number of chapters they found in their life stories was eleven, although it varied among individuals. Henner recommends eight to fifteen chapters.

Finding Other Life-Story Themes

Some meaningful memories do not fit neatly into a chronological order but still have a common theme. If I recall hiking trips, for example, there is no particular connection between them other than they involved hiking, so they don't neatly arrange into a chapter. Nonetheless, it is satisfying to revisit them, and once I think of one trip, another is easily brought to mind. This is also true for the artist who thinks back to the creations she has worked on, or the woodworker and his projects, or the baseball fan's all-time favorite games. Topics that might be associated with memories like these are shown in the box on the next page. By identifying such areas, you open up opportunities for pleasant reminiscing.

Personal Mementos

Memory recall requires memory cues, and mementos can be especially effective—pictures from a vacation, a high school yearbook, a coffee mug made by a friend—all can be powerful reminders. The traditional way to collect and organize small mementos is the scrapbook. People keep them

---

Possibilities for Life Chapters

Places you've lived	Jobs	Children
High school	College	Grandchildren
Brothers / sisters	Childhood	Marriage
Parents	Hobbies	Divorce

Other Memorable Themes

Turning points in life	Friendships	Pets
Lessons from life	Outdoor adventures	Romances
Vacations	Family events	Mentors
Sporting activities	Spiritual experiences	Great meals
Work projects	Collections	Cars

for various reasons—to document events, to chronicle the past, to create pleasing displays—but every item carefully glued in place is a memory cue for an event meaningful to the scrapbooker, and this makes scrapbooks potent aids to autobiographical memory in the same way photo albums are. When you select a memento for inclusion, you identify it as something worth remembering. As you handle the object to secure it on the page, relevant memories come to mind, making them stronger.

Other sources of memorabilia also provide strong cues. Hearing a bar of music associated with a happy time, preparing stuffing for Thanksgiving dinner, smelling roses can all bring back memories that would be inaccessible otherwise. Studies have identified jewelry, stuffed animals, letters, and diaries as helpful cues for women. Men showed better reminiscence to sports equipment, cars, and trophies of past accomplishments. Memorabilia also play a role in the lives of people with HSAM—they are avid collectors and organizers of bits and pieces from the past.

The Act of Remembering

Suppose you have chosen a memory to explore. How might you recall it to get the richest experience? For example, say I want to remember a trip my wife and I took to San Francisco. Memory expert Dominic O'Brien recommends starting with a specific detail and working outward from there. The first detail that comes to my mind is the registration desk at the hotel. As I bring that into focus, other details start returning—the pleasant woman who checked us in, riding in the antique elevator, the four-poster bed. More memories easily follow—climbing steep sidewalks, friendly people we met, the smell of the waterfront. As one memory cues the next, I re-create the experience.

The way you picture memories as you recall them can affect how vivid they seem to you—the most powerful approach is to recall the experience from an "internal" perspective. This means I remember the cable car ride as it looked to me through my own eyes rather than picturing the ride as it would appear to an external camera recording the scene. Marilu Henner reports she always remembers this way, but most of us can't do this with all our memories. Instead, our memories are a mix of internal and external perspectives. Both viewpoints are seen in a memory recalled by a twenty-one-year-old undergraduate:

> I see myself dancing at a party at the university. I remember my clothes and my legs (the way they moved). Suddenly I am "inside my own body" looking out. A guy I know a little walks by and says as he passes, "You look good today."

She began with an external perspective but switched to an internal perspective as the memory unfolds. If she maintains that perspective, she will find that the emotions she remembers are more intense and the sensory details richer than they would be from an external viewpoint.

For recent memories, you will find an internal perspective relatively easy and natural to adopt. Older memories, which can be weaker and less detailed, may come to mind only from an external perspective, probably because they have faded to the point where they no longer have the sensory richness needed for an internal view. Forcing a memory like this into an internal perspective won't be a benefit. But when you can recall a memory readily from either an internal or external vantage point, the internal perspective will be a richer experience.

It's helpful to keep in mind that a specific memory doesn't always have to be recalled in the same way—a fresh perspective can sometimes provide a new take on an old memory. Henner identified four ways to re-create an experience. In the "horizontal" approach, the memory is recalled like a linear story—we arrive in San Francisco at the airport, take a taxi, check in, and so on. She uses the analogy of a DVD video for this kind of recall, cuing up one scene after the other as you move through the event. The "vertical" approach looks closely at one part of the experience—the lunch we had on the pier with the view, the table, the server, what we ordered, and the feelings of that moment. A "mushroom" approach starts with the San Francisco memory and uses it as a cue for wherever it leads, such as a time on the Atlantic City waterfront. A fourth type of retrieval is to capitalize on spontaneous recollections when they occur, such as when a random sight or sound brings to mind a part of the San Francisco trip. Usually we pay little attention to such involuntary memories, but when the situation permits, we can choose to hold them in consciousness, let them develop, and thus bring back the experience.

As you work on improving reminiscing, you will find the three structured retrieval strategies of Chapter 5 helpful. The mnemonic from that chapter, shown in the figure below, can help in remembering them. The "shotgun" strategy uses free association to find retrieval cues that activate other memories. The "return to the scene" strategy takes you back to the setting where the memory occurred to mentally re-create it and look for memory cues. The "wait-and-try-again" strategy allows time to pass between retrieval efforts. It can be surprising and rewarding to discover just what can come back when you stumble on the right cue after using one of these techniques. But don't overdo efforts to dredge up long-lost memories. If you struggle and struggle to remember, you can find yourself "recalling" a compelling false memory that never happened, an invention that you inadvertently created by overzealous efforts. So, give these techniques a chance, but if they don't produce the memory you were seeking, move on to other memories that can be more readily recalled. These are more likely to be valid reflections of the past.

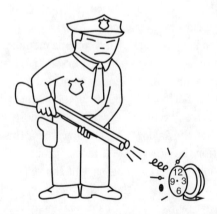

A mnemonic for recall strategies: the shotgun approach, the return to the scene approach (the cop), and the wait and try again approach (the clock).

In the Memory Lab: Creating a Habit of Reminiscing

If you want to spend more time reflecting on your life, you could follow the lead of people with HSAM and develop a habit of reminiscing. Marilu Henner speaks for all of them when she says, "I know that part of the reason I have such a strong memory is because I spent my entire life instinctively reviewing my past." In this installment of the Memory Lab, we look at the mechanics of establishing a habit of autobiographical reminiscing. Doing so gives me the opportunity to discuss habits and their creation, which is useful knowledge for any practitioner of the memory arts.

Habits are a special kind of memory similar to skills, the topic of the last chapter, but with their own characteristics. Reading is a skill; sitting down with the newspaper at breakfast is a habit. Both are behavioral sequences established by repetition, but skills are complex, flexible, and directed toward a specific goal like understanding the printed word. Habits are simpler, more situation specific, and less flexible. In fact, if I am eating breakfast in a restaurant, I don't feel a strong need to have the newspaper before me because my newspaper habit is connected to breakfast at my own kitchen table.

Because habits are automatic routines, we do them without conscious effort. This makes them particularly useful when we want to establish a desirable new behavior. If reminiscing can become a habit, it will be activated whenever you are in the triggering situation. Once that happens, you'll enter what Henner calls an "autobiographical state of mind," where you begin thinking about the past. This prompts you to take it from there and examine an aspect of your life.

As the diagram on the next page shows, a habit begins with a triggering cue. Next the behavior occurs—in this case, reminiscing. The last step is a positive outcome that acts like a reward to encourage the behavior in the future. Habits are established by repeating the sequence over and over.

Finding a Trigger

What you're looking for is a specific setting where you can pause to reflect on your life, one where you can have a few private minutes to

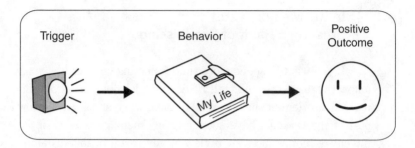

The three-step sequence that is repeated over and over to create a habit.

reminisce. People with HSAM report habitually reviewing their past in situations such as when shaving, when going to sleep, when awakening in the morning, when stuck in traffic, when waiting for an appointment, or when writing in a journal. The most powerful triggers are those that have the same sensory cues each time—the same sights, sounds, smells. An example is Jill Price blow-drying her hair in the morning, a trigger that initiates her habit of reviewing memories from previous days with the same date.

Carrying Out the Behavior

You will need topics to reminisce about, and it will help at this stage if you have them picked out ahead of time. Consider developing a list of possibilities such as specific life chapters or themes or events. Each day you can select one from the list. The amount of time you spend reminiscing is your call, but I recommend that you keep it short at first, just a few minutes.

Experiencing a Positive Outcome

For most people, the reward for reminiscing is built into the process. Reviewing the past to understand the path you've followed or to solve a problem is usually satisfying. Even when the memories are unpleasant, you may be able to adopt a perspective that gives them a different, more constructive meaning. Here is Marilu Henner's take on this:

. . . try to think of bad memories with the same appreciation you have when going through an archive box you haven't touched in ten years. Each item that comes out tells a story, and seeing it many years later gives new insight to how you understood it when it actually happened. A current perspective gives you a more objective understanding. You begin to clearly recognize why you made certain choices and how you would respond differently to similar circumstances in the future.

Overall, you should expect most of your reminiscing to be a good experience. This is what makes reminiscing constructive and why it seems to be associated with well-being. A positive outcome to reminiscing is also important at this stage because it serves as a reward that facilitates habit formation by encouraging repetition.

How Long Will It Take?

A habit is considered completely formed when it becomes automatic. You'll know when this happens: The trigger situation will put you into an autobiographical frame of mind in which you will want to reminisce. Unfortunately, you can't know in advance just how many repetitions it will take. In one study, students undertook to develop simple habits like eating a piece of fruit with lunch or running fifteen minutes before dinner. On average, it took sixty-six days to develop the behaviors into automatic habits. Individual students, though, were all over the map, ranging from eighteen days to 254 days! The moral is to be patient if you want a true habit to develop.

13

The PARIS Mnemonics

What if you could find versatile and practical ways to boost your memory in everyday situations like remembering shopping lists, errands, appointments, travel directions, and even speeches and presentations? It turns out you can do just that by tapping in to a small group of tried and proven mnemonic strategies that have wide applicability and are worthy additions to the repertoire of any mnemonist. These five techniques are named below and paired with an image associated with their acronym, PARIS. You have seen some of them in the Memory Lab sections of previous chapters, where I introduced them as techniques for remembering material from the chapter. Now let's take a closer look at these and related mnemonic templates.

Peg Words

Here is a mental notepad that will help you retain any information that can take the form of a list. I call on it often—it helps me remember what I want

Peg Words
Acrostics and Acronyms
Rhymes and Rhythm
Imagery
Stories

to get done before a trip, items to buy at the store, commitments I make at a staff meeting, or tasks and ideas that come to me in the middle of the night. Most often, it is information I will need for only a day or two. The peg words are a set of concrete objects you associate with the items you want to remember, words you can readily retrieve at a later time. The mnemonic is based on an easy-to-remember set of rhymes:

One is a Bun	Six is Sticks
Two is a Shoe	Seven is Heaven
Three is a Tree	Eight is a Gate
Four is a Door	Nine is Wine
Five is a Hive	Ten is a Hen

Once you've established the peg words in your memory—which won't take long—you can use them to remember any list up to ten items by associating the first item on the list with a bun, the second with a shoe, the third with a tree, and so on. The key to making this work is creating dramatic, distinctive imagery of the memory items interacting with the peg words. So, if you want to pick up onions, a tomato, and celery at the store, you first create an image of onions and a bun—perhaps an onion sandwich with a huge pile of sliced onions inside the bun. Next you move to the tomato and try to get something going with the shoe. You might visualize a shoe that has just stepped on a ripe tomato, making a yucky mess. You could associate the celery with a tree by imagining a magnificent giant celery tree.

Once you're at the store, reciting the rhyme—"one is a bun; two is a shoe; three is a tree"—will bring back the images and trigger memory for the items. Research studies show what will be clear to anyone who tries it: If your images create a good connection between the peg words and the list items, the mnemonic will serve you exceedingly well. And you needn't worry that you might confuse the new images with those left over from the last list you memorized. This just doesn't happen in practice. The newest association will be the one you recall—it's similar to parking your car when you go to work. Where you left your car yesterday doesn't confuse you about where you parked today.

Its Two Strengths

The peg word strategy excels in two areas where mnemonics can aid memory. First, it helps organize material to make it easier to retrieve when you need it. The peg words technique uses our well-learned ability to count as its organizing principle—as you mentally run through the digits, each item on your grocery list is cued in turn. Second, peg words can improve the memorability of individual memory items with better encoding. Here again, peg words get high marks. When you use imagery to connect "onions" on your grocery list with "bun" as a peg word, the odds of remembering the onions shoot up. As you will see, not all the PARIS mnemonics are equally strong in both organizing and encoding, and this makes the peg word strategy noteworthy. It is a simple, powerful, elegant way to remember a list.

Its Weakness

Like any of the imagery methods, this strategy is more difficult to use when the material is not easy to visualize. Consider a to-do list that includes "check out insurance." You decide to put "insurance" on your peg word list, but no concrete image comes to mind to represent it. A way around the problem is the substitute word approach. You look for a concrete word that *sounds* close enough to "insurance" to suggest it—perhaps "insect." Now you create an image associating the substitute word with a peg word. Later when you use the peg word to recall "insect," its sound helps you remember "insurance." We saw this technique used to remember names in Chapter 7. Substitute words work, but they add a complication that takes effort to overcome.

Peg Word Variations

Rhyming words are only one of several ways to set up a useful peg word system. In fact, we saw an alternate approach in Chapter 10, when we looked at the "major system" for remembering numbers. That system also associates concrete objects with specific digits, but the objects are selected based on the letters in their names. This gave pairings like 1—tie, 2—hen, and 3—ma. Their key features are the consonants t, n, and m, the established codes for the digits 1, 2, and 3. Vowels and other sounds were added to create concrete words. The major system can readily give a concrete word for each number from 0 to 99, as we saw in that chapter. Some mnemonists use this system to remember lists in the same way I use the rhyming peg words. It has the advantage that it can handle more than ten items. Another possibility is to construct peg words from the alphabet with pairings like

A—ape, B—boy, and C—cat. Any of these systems will work, and it comes down to personal preference. I reserve the major system for remembering numbers and use the rhyming peg word system for remembering lists. I find I can recall the rhyming words more rapidly with less effort than the words of the other systems.

Acronyms and Acrostics

You'll recall these two mnemonic forms from the Memory Lab segments of earlier chapters. Called "first-letter mnemonics," for obvious reasons, they provide useful ways to organize and remember items on a list. Unlike the peg word method, these mnemonics work as well with abstract words as they do with concrete ones. That is why I chose an acronym (PARIS) to encode this chapter's five mnemonic techniques. We saw another example in Chapter 8 to encode three ways to strengthen prospective memory (ICE)—which refers to Implementation intentions, Cue imagery, and Exaggerated importance.

Acronyms are usually short, typically no more than five or six letters. It helps if they are pronounceable, and the best ones, like PARIS and ICE, form recognizable words. Other well-known acronyms are HOMES to encode the Great Lakes (Huron, Ontario, Michigan, Erie, and Superior) and RAPPOS to recall the First Amendment protections of the U.S. Constitution (religion, assembly, petition, press, opinion, and speech).

The RAPPOS mnemonic is interesting in that it includes "opinion," a protection not listed in the First Amendment—it's covered as free speech. The inventor of the acronym probably added it to encourage pronunciation of both Ps, something that might not happen if the acronym were RAPPS.

Acrostics are conceptually similar to acronyms, but their strength is that they form a meaningful phrase, and this allows them to support longer lists such as the Romantic Dragon acrostic of Chapter 4—"**R**omantic **D**ragons **E**at **V**egetables **A**nd **P**refer **O**nions"—which cues seven principles for strengthening memories: Retention intention, Deep processing, Elaboration, Visualization, Association, Practice, and Organization. An equivalent seven-letter acronym (REDAVOP, perhaps) is cumbersome and more difficult to remember. Even for shorter lists, an acrostic can be a good choice if the only available acronym is unpronounceable or awkward. That was the case in Chapter 7 with the mnemonic for remembering how to learn names and faces: Find a Feature, Listen, Say it, and Practice. The acrostic "Friendly Llamas Seek People" is better than the awkward acronym FLSP.

As acrostics get longer and longer, they lead to ever more clumsy sentences. Consider this fifteen-word acrostic for chemistry's Electromotive Series: "Poorly Canned Sausages Make A Zulu Ill. Therefore Let Highly Clever Men Slay Good Pigs" (Potassium, Calcium, Sodium, Magnesium, Aluminum, Zinc, Iron, Tin, Lead, Hydrogen, Copper, Mercury, Silver, Gold, Platinum). The complex acrostic is definitely easier to remember than the chemical list, but it will take some effort and rehearsal to master. The acrostic's creator was wise to develop it as two relatively short sentences, a kindness for those who must learn it. In general, as the length of the memory list increases, the acrostic becomes more and more contorted. At some point, it becomes prudent to move to what is known as a "memory palace," an approach I will describe in the next chapter.

A strength of acronyms and acrostics is that by encoding the first letters of the items in a word or phrase, they give the list an organization that helps you remember it. An added benefit is that they let you know how many items you must recall and when recall is complete. Their weakness is that they don't provide much help in making the items more memorable— they assume the first letter of each one will be enough to cue its memory. This may or may not be true. Go back to the acronym RAPPOS and see if it succeeds in cueing the protections of the First Amendment. If you missed some, you are not alone. It's not that the specific protections are difficult words or that the protections are unfamiliar; the problem is that they have not been associated together well enough to allow the single-letter cues to retrieve them. For many of us, this acronym can only work if we strengthen and associate memories for the protections so that we could recall them even with the acronym's relatively weak cue. This will require practicing the mnemonic until the protections easily come to mind.

Rhymes and Rhythms

Wonder which way to turn that screw? Say, "Righty tighty, lefty loosey." Come upon a person in shock? Have the person lie down and think, "If the face is red, raise the head. If the face is pale, raise the tail." Planning on serious partying? Keep in mind that "Beer on whiskey, very risky; whiskey on beer, never fear."

Rhymes and rhythms have long been used as mnemonic aids and for good reason—both are effective memory cues. To see why, take another look at the Henry limerick from Chapter 9.

Henry

There once was a boy named Henry
Who tried to improve his memory.
He practiced facts that he faced
With retrieval well spaced,
And found his recall exemplary.

Once you recall that easy first line you are well on your way, because the second line has to conform to it by (1) rhyming with "Henry," (2) adhering to the standard limerick rhythm, and (3) making sense. It is as if three pieces of a jigsaw puzzle are suddenly in place—rhyme, rhythm, and meaning—and the next piece must interlock with them. As memory researcher David Rubin pointed out, these three features drastically narrow the possibilities for what can come next, and this allows the memory system to more easily find the words that follow. Rhyme, rhythm, and meaning function as both memory cues and memory constraints. This is why we find mnemonic structures like rhyming maxims or limericks easy to remember.

Rhyming mnemonics always have a rhythm that emphasizes the rhyming words. In the Henry limerick, it's

There ONCE was a boy named HENRY
Who TRIED to improve his MEMORY.

It is this intonation pattern that allows rhyming to work well as a memory retrieval strategy. Normally we don't search our memory for rhymes. We can easily do it—bye, sky, high, die—but only if we intend to. The contribution of the sing-song rhythm is that it emphasizes words that must rhyme. This signals "rhyming mode," cueing the memory system to search for appropriate matches.

Rhythm can work as a memory cue even without rhymes, and it has played a role in extraordinary memory feats. During the age of the Roman Empire, it was not unknown for people to memorize the entire *Aeneid*, an epic poem of almost 10,000 lines written by Virgil in about 20 B.C. The distinctive rhythm of the poem's lines, a sound pattern known as dactylic hexameter, provided the structure that made such a massive undertaking possible. In the present day, there are millions of Muslims, called Hafiz, who have committed the entire *Quran* to memory. This work, written in Arabic, contains more than 6,000 verses and 80,000 words. As in the *Aeneid*, its lines do not rhyme. What is especially impressive is that many Hafiz do not speak Arabic, and therefore the words they memorize have no meaning to them. Their effort begins with learning to pronounce Arabic words to bring out the rhythm of the *Quran*'s passages. That rhythm becomes their principal memory aid as they laboriously master verse after verse during perhaps three years of study.

Rhyme and rhythm are unusual among the mnemonic forms in this chapter because they can be used for purposes other than remembering a list. They facilitate memory for all sorts of verbatim text. The text might contain a principle, like the Henry limerick, or a suggestion, like the mnemonic for turning a screw, or it can be a major work like the *Quran*. Rhyme and rhythm stand as a container for any verbal content a memoirist wants to embed in it.

Imagery

Imagery is, of course, everywhere in the memory arts, and we have encountered it often in this book. Here we look at a fundamental, imagery-based technique that is the simplest and most basic of all mnemonic strategies. Called the "link method," it helps you remember a list by creating a series of visual associations between pairs of memory items, building a chain of associations that eventually includes the entire list. We saw an example in Chapter 11, where I used the link method to remember topics for a lecture.

Because of its simplicity, memory teachers often use it to demonstrate the power of mnemonics to new students. Harry Lorayne, the great memory performer and memory trainer, was a master at this. Students at his workshops were barely settled into their seats when he had them remembering a list. The following selection, taken from one of his many books, captures his approach. Here Lorayne talks his readers through using the link method to retain this list of objects: envelope, airplane, wristwatch, pill, insect, wallet, bathtub, and shoe.

> Starting with **envelope/airplane**, begin by visualizing an envelope. Then mentally "attach" that to airplane: a gigantic envelope is flying like an airplane;

an airplane is licking and sealing a gigantic envelope; millions of envelopes are boarding or disembarking an airplane; you're trying to stuff an airplane into an envelope. You need only one picture, so select one I've just suggested, or one you've thought of yourself and *see* it. . . .

Airplane/Wristwatch. The new thing, wristwatch, must be brought to mind by airplane. Can you see yourself wearing a large airplane on your wrist instead of a watch? Or maybe there is a gigantic wristwatch around each wing of the airplane, or a gigantic wristwatch is flying like an airplane. . . . *See* one of those pictures in your mind.

On he goes, pair after pair, with nonstop patter to help his students create graphic visual images that link each pair on the list. After he finishes, he has them remember the items, which they find they can do with relative ease. Then, in a final flourish, he challenges students to recall the list backwards. Lo and behold, they discover that this too was easy. With his audience amazed and motivated, Lorayne is ready to move on to the next workshop topic.

The link method is well suited for Lorayne's purposes because it requires little preparation. There are no peg words to memorize, no acrostics to invent, just imaginative associations to connect pairs of objects. Once the associations are in place you can move up or down the list item by item.

A weakness of the link method is that it creates a chain of associations only as good as its weakest link. If you forget one of them, you can become stymied. And if you forget the first item on the list, you may find yourself with a catastrophic failure in which you can't recall any of the items. The lesson here is to rehearse the list well enough to establish the links securely in your memory. What I do if I have even the slightest worry about remembering the first item is create a starting link to make sure I can bring it to mind. I use an image of a boat anchor and associate it with the first list item.

On the mnemonic scorecard, the peg word system is superior to the link method because it doesn't have the "weakest link" problem. If you forget a word in the peg word system, nothing else is compromised; you just move on. But despite its shortcoming, the link method has advantages. It is easy to apply—there's no need to bother with mentally manipulating peg words. It also is particularly useful when all you want to remember is the next item on a list—say when you must remember the next topic in a speech or the next product on a shopping list. With the link method, your recall effort goes right to the one association relevant at that moment, the association that gets you to the next item on the list.

Stories

For centuries, the collective memory of entire cultures was maintained by stories told by one generation to the next. Stories are natural mnemonic devices. They work well because they play to the strengths of the memory system. They are based on meaning; they organize the material; they encourage deep processing; they contain elaborations, and they provide associations. These strengths no doubt explain why stories are so often trusted with important information—the wisdom of Aesop, the parables of the bible, the cultural lessons of folk tales.

The mnemonic benefits of the story can be harnessed simply by adding a narrative to forgettable information, and it can be used in conjunction with any other memory aid. Suppose you are using the peg word mnemonic to remember a shopping list, and you come to an association between "bun" and "onions." If your image of an onion sandwich on a bun seems uninspired, you could invent a story to pump it up: "This sandwich," you might say to yourself, "has been entered in a national food competition for a huge prize. It features extra sweet onions that are sure to please the judges." A quick, fanciful story like this can go a long way to ensure that the image will be available when you need it.

Stories can also be used as a primary memory aid. We saw an example of this in Chapter 10 in the way that Chao Lu memorized the first 61,890 digits of *pi*. He remembered each pair of digits as a concrete object, and then he wove a group of objects into a story that he connected to other stories. He repeated the process until he had the long chain of stories that allowed him to retain that massive number of digits.

We can use the story approach in the same way by creating a narrative around items we want to remember. To remember a shopping list—onions, tomato, celery, milk, and bread—you can create a plot to pull the items together. Here is one possibility.

> An **onion** walks into a bar and sits next to an overripe **tomato**. The barkeep, a tall stalk of **celery**, comes over, and the **onion** orders **milk**. Celery slides the drink down the bar. The **tomato** sneers, "milk in a bar?" and continues to eat her **bread,** carefully dunking each bite in her martini.

It helps to visualize a story as well as verbalizing it, and a rehearsal or two is always a good idea. Research supports the story method as an effective mnemonic. In one study, college students remembered six times as many words after weaving them into a story as they did without a story. The technique has been especially successful when the material was tested after periods longer than a few days. It has also been shown to work with older adults and may be easier for them to use than other mnemonics.

A story achieves its memory benefit by using narrative to organize memory material and provide memory cues to recall it. A coherent story carries out these two functions well. But like the link method, the organization and cueing are provided by the memory material itself, so if you forget one thing, there can be a domino effect.

Stories work best when the list of memory items is not too long. Chao Lu held each story segment to about five memory items. That was also the size of my grocery list example. Imagine expanding that story to accommodate fifteen items—it would take a significant investment of time and effort, and the final product would likely be a convoluted tale, one with real possibilities for slippage. But when the lists are not too long, say, ten or fewer items, the story mnemonic is an entertaining and satisfying way to exercise the memory arts. When I ask students in my memory classes to try different mnemonics for lists and pick a favorite, the story mnemonic is always among their top choices.

A Final Thought

The PARIS mnemonics are general-purpose memory strategies for use with any memory material you can plug into them. They let you forgo written notes and electronic devices for routine memory needs and instead engage your wits and your knowledge of memory. For example, do you really need a written list when you go to the store? Wouldn't it be rewarding to go to the store without a written list and still come home with every item you intended to buy? And couldn't you just call up that to-do list with a PARIS strategy? What about the questions you want to ask the doctor? Or the topics you'll use to enliven that obligatory phone call to your mother-in-law?

The PARIS mnemonics can also be used to pump up natural memory. For a business presentation, you could retain the points you want to make in a list mnemonic—Introductory remark → The problem → Option 1 → Option 2 → Recommendation. By picking a concrete word to cue each point and linking them together, you can run over the presentation easily before the meeting. When you go to make the points, you will probably not need the mnemonic, because the rehearsals will have put the information at your fingertips and prepared your natural memory to perform well. This strategy is useful in any setting—presentations, job interviews, sales pitches—where you need to speak without notes or PowerPoint.

Of course, you don't have to use mnemonics to retain the kinds of information I've talked about—a pad of sticky notes and a pencil will get you through all those situations. But the PARIS strategies are rewarding exercises because they give you, as a recreational practitioner of the memory arts, a chance to accept a mental challenge and meet it. They allow you to step away from ubiquitous smart phones and iPads and exercise your mental resources. The reward is not only personal satisfaction but also the knowledge that you are putting to good use your most sophisticated mental processes—working memory, attention, top-down control, self-discipline, and self-reliance.

There is still one more technique to add to your mnemonic repertoire, one more option for holding on to slippery information. Like the PARIS mnemonics, it is applicable to memory material that can be put in the form of a list. This final strategy is rightfully considered the pinnacle of the ancient memory arts, one taught to students for centuries and extolled by luminaries from Cicero and Thomas Aquinas right up to Joshua Foer and Dominic O'Brien. This remarkable method of memory enhancement is the topic of the next chapter.

In the Memory Lab:
Test Driving the Paris Mnemonics

The best way to get a feel for the PARIS mnemonics is to try them out. Except for the rhyme/rhythm format, they are well suited for remembering not only shopping lists and to-do lists, but also appointments, passwords, and directions. Your test drive can start with random, concrete words, and I've provided the five short lists on the facing page for that purpose. In each case, the goal should be to use one of the mnemonic formats to retain the list for a day or two. As you carry this out, enjoy your successes but also pay attention to slippages. Often you can learn a lot about the practicalities of specific mnemonics by trying to understand why you forgot something. Now the lists:

Peg words: meadow, stork, elbow, package, fox
Acronym: organ, steeple, knuckle, basin, eagle
Acrostic: prune, sword, lemon, spoke, statue
Imagery (link method): reed, nail, road, urn, wine
Story: edge, dairy, rattle, monarch, brim

14

The Memory Palace

Between 2001 and 2006, Andrew Card Jr. was the chief of staff for President George W. Bush. It was Card's responsibility to manage the president's daily schedule on a 24/7 basis, doing whatever was needed, from arranging key meetings to knowing the time of the president's next haircut appointment. It was a high-stakes job filled with endless, crucial, and not-so-crucial details. Card held the position longer than any of his predecessors in the last fifty years.

If you assume that Card designed and maintained an elaborate finely tuned filing system or a computerized spreadsheet to keep track of his responsibilities, you're mistaken. Reports say he seldom took notes at meetings and kept his desk clean, almost empty, with no paper in evidence. In fact, Andrew Card's notes and reminders and schedules were all in his head. He managed his pressure-cooker job almost solely by means of a remarkable mnemonic system called a "memory palace," the contents of which he juggled constantly as tasks, issues, and people came and went.

A memory palace is a group of fixed, well-known locations that one can easily imagine—say rooms in your home or different spots along a street in your neighborhood. It is often called the "Method of Loci" ("places" in Latin). To use a palace, you create visual associations between specific places and the information to be remembered—so, you could retain a grocery list by imagining each item at a different place in your palace—in the linen closet, on the dining room table, in the bathtub. Later, at the store, you mentally go to each place, discover the images you've created, and remember the items.

Card's memory palace was the kitchen of his boyhood home. Its features served as mental storage locations—the stove, the countertop, cabinets, and other kitchen furnishings. The information he stored there was more complex than a grocery list, but the principle was the same. Each fact or task was represented by a mental image associated with a specific place. A 2005 *Washington Post* story described the memory palace in operation.

> When tackling matters of top priority, Card [imagines standing] at the stove, working his "front and back burners." Intelligence reform is cooking this morning. He needs to call several people: 9/11 commission Chairmen Tom Kean and Lee Hamilton, Reps Duncan Hunter and James Sensenbrenner, and House Speaker Dennis Hastert. They are "on my right Front Burner," he says.
>
> "Then I shift gears to my left front burner, which is second most important," Card says. He will help the president hire a Cabinet secretary, then move to his right rear burner (hiring White House staff for the second term). "I do all that in my kitchen," Card says. "Now the things I want to put off for a long time, I put in the freezer. But then I can go to my freezer and generally remember things that I put there a long time ago." He will store matters that were resolved or tabled yesterday in a cupboard.

In an interview with me in 2009, he elaborated on his palace, describing other locations, each designed to serve a bustling office that needed to handle an ever-changing mix of ongoing work, new demands, crises, and important people. He used the oven for situations that needed to stay warm for a day or two before they could be resolved; the microwave held projects that needed to be done quickly, and the sink was for messes that needed cleaning up. When a memory item was no longer needed, Card took its memory image to the disposal and "let go" of it. He said he always paused before putting anything in the disposal, asking himself if he really wanted to get rid of it because he would almost certainly forget it once he let it go.

Card told me he seldom took notes at meetings, deciding instead what he wanted to remember and mentally putting that in the proper spot in the kitchen. Information he needed during the meeting he would retrieve from the kitchen. Periodically during the day he would "clean the kitchen" by mentally running through it, updating this, acting on that, and refreshing the information stored there. Card had used this system for decades.

Card's interest in memory palaces began in high school when he had a chance encounter with a memory performer who told him about the procedure. That conversation created a lifelong interest in mnemonic technique.

Soon he was applying the methods to his schoolwork and his afterschool job at a fast-food restaurant. The mental challenge of mnemonics appealed to him, and his skill increased, eventually carrying over to his duties at the White House. Did he think his natural memory was unusually good? I asked him. He said that he did not believe so. Instead, he attributed his remarkable ability to mental discipline in maintaining his kitchen. It was a process that was engaging and rewarding to him.

The Method of Loci in Antiquity

The Method of Loci that Card made such good use of has been a valued memory aid for more than two millennia. Legend has it that it was discovered in Greece about 500 B.C. by a renowned poet, Simonides, also known as "the honey tongued." Cicero, writing four centuries later in about 50 B.C., gave the best surviving account of the event. It seems that a nobleman planning a feast in his own honor contracted with Simonides to write an ode for the occasion extolling the nobleman's greatness. When it was read at the feast, the nobleman was taken aback by a section devoted to the exploits of two youthful gods, Castor and Pollux. Incensed, the nobleman told Simonides he would pay only half the agreed-upon price and that he should collect the other half from the two gods. Shortly thereafter, a servant told Simonides that there were two young men outside waiting to see him. But when he went out he found no one. At that very moment, the roof collapsed, killing all and mangling them so badly that identification was impossible. Simonides, however, was able to remember who was sitting where around the table by picturing the scene. That visual memory allowed relatives to claim the bodies. Later Simonides reflected on the experience and formulated the Method of Loci, based on the principle that an organized set of known places could help a person remember anything associated with them.

Simonides lived at the beginning of the classical Greek period when architecture flourished and democratic forms of government were emerging. Education became more valued, literacy more common, and written works more available. One might think that moving from an oral to a written culture would reduce memory demands, not increase them. But classical archaeologist Jocelyn Penny Small suggests that writing in fact had the opposite effect, creating a need for memory skill and a market for the memory arts. To understand why, consider the nature of written texts at the time.

When we think of "writing," we imagine what printed words look like on a page like this one, but what you are reading is writing that has been refined by innovations unknown to the Greeks and Romans. They experienced writing in a form that came to be called *scriptio continua,* used until about A.D. 1000, in which there were no spaces or punctuation between words, sentences, or paragraphs. The next paragraph appears in *scriptio continua* format and then is followed by the same words presented in the modern format. *Scriptio continua* was usually read aloud syllable by syllable, not word by word, and the reader listened to the sounds as he spoke them, using sound along with the letters on the page to decode the message. The manuscript itself was a long scroll. A major work like the *Iliad,* which spans more than 400 pages in a modern book, comprised twenty-four scrolls. There were no chapter titles, no headings, no table of contents, no index, and sometimes no manuscript title. Pity the poor reader who forgot a point and returned to the scroll to check it. Indeed, far from rendering memory skill obsolete, the written word made it essential. It would be many centuries before such niceties as spacing between words, upper and lower case, punctuation, paragraphing, headings, and consistent spelling came into wide use.

```
THUSITWASTHATSIMONIDESDISCOVERYPROVIDEDATECHNIQUETHAT
HADPRACTICALVALUEFORSTUDENTSANDSCHOLARSITWASPICKED
UPANDDISSEMINATEDBYTHESOPHISTSAGROUPOFITINERANT
INTELLECTUALSWHOTUTOREDSTUDENTSINPHILOSOPHYSPEAKING
ANDWRITINGARISTOTLEPROVIDEDANADDITIONALBOOSTFORTHE
METHODBYENDORSINGITANDITISLIKELYTHATHEWASSKILLEDIN
ITSUSE
```

(Thus it was that Simonides's discovery provided a technique that had practical value for students and scholars. It was picked up and disseminated by the Sophists, a group of itinerant intellectuals who tutored students in philosophy, speaking, and writing. Aristotle [350 b.c.] provided an additional boost for the method by endorsing it, and it is likely that he was skilled in its use.)

When Greece was added to the Roman Empire in 146 B.C., memory strategies spread to the West and became part of a standard curriculum taught to privileged sons of the wealthy on their way to high-status careers. The memory skills they learned benefited them in more ways than just as a study aid because memory ability itself was highly valued by the Romans. Its signature demonstration was in public oratory. Standout orators like Cicero were widely admired, and crowds were dazzled by their ability to deliver eloquent presentations without notes. The Method of Loci provided support for these deliveries and more. Memory scholar Mary Carruthers believes that the great orators used their memory palaces creatively to analyze complex situations, invent winning arguments, and handle objections from opponents.

Matteo Ricci

Although the concept of a memory palace is straightforward, many details about how memory palaces were actually used are elusive. What role did they play in education? How long was the information remembered? In what settings other than oratory were they useful? Most ancient descriptions of memory techniques are general and brief because it was assumed that their application was common knowledge. There is a notable exception, however: a sixteenth-century priest named Matteo Ricci. Although he was many centuries removed from the heyday of the Roman era, he had mastered the same memory arts and even studied from texts written in Cicero's day. His story provides insights into real-world applications of these memory aids. Before I tell it, though, let me fill in a few developments from the intervening years.

The classic memory arts—visualization, organization, and association, along with the Method of Loci—continued to be taught and practiced in the Roman Empire until it collapsed around the year 500. Massive upheaval followed as great cities fell into disarray, the educational infrastructure vanished, and literacy declined dramatically. Among the casualties were the memory arts, which disappeared from use. Surprisingly, though, in the thirteenth century, the arts were revived when scholarly monks discovered long-lost Roman texts that described them. One of these monks was the great Catholic theologian Thomas Aquinas, a Dominican friar born in 1225, who studied the ancient works, became expert in the memory arts, and used them to advantage in writing his influential works. Thomas came to the conclusion that memory skill was important to a Christian seeking salvation because "memory of many things" is a prerequisite to wise moral choices. With his endorsement, the Method of Loci became not just a practical skill but one considered morally virtuous. The Dominicans, and later the Jesuits, taught Thomist views widely and helped spread the use of the memory arts among the educated elite. Well before the sixteenth century, training in memory was common in the schools and colleges of these religious orders.

Matteo Ricci, born in Italy in 1552, received that training. Later the memory skills he learned contributed to his success as a Jesuit missionary to China. When historian Jonathan Spence wrote *The Memory Palace of Matteo Ricci*, his remarkable book about Ricci's life and times, he unearthed many details about Ricci's training and life that offer revealing glimpses of the mnemonic practices of his day.

Ricci joined the Jesuits in 1571 and attended the prestigious Jesuit College of Rome for much of his training. The Jesuits, founded in 1540, took pride in being at the forefront of the intellectual issues of the day and prepared students for this distinction with heavy workloads in the humanities, theology, science, and mathematics. Training in memory was an integral part of their education, and Ricci had access to expert memory instruction. Spence believes one of his memory teachers may have been Francesco Panigarola, who was said to be able "to roam across a hundred thousand memory images, each in its own fixed space." Ricci likely constructed many memory palaces as part of his education, something like a memory city with different structures to hold different subjects.

Ricci's memory palaces probably had varied forms. Some were certainly buildings such as the grand cathedrals he would have known, each with many locations within its walls for memory images. Other palaces were probably familiar routes he traveled around Rome or his home city of Macerata. The landmarks along these journeys would have been ideal memory locations. Some of his palaces may have been figurines in the form of statues or images of fictional characters. The drawing on the next page, which dates from 1533, is an example. It is a personification of "grammar," one of the seven liberal arts Ricci would have studied. Historian Frances Yates, whose book, *The Art of Memory*, was my source for this drawing, believes that figures like this were in use in Roman times and in the Middle Ages as variations on the Method of Loci. The mysterious-looking objects and lettering around Gramatica are thought to be memory cues for grammatical principles, each one occupying a specific location in the drawing,

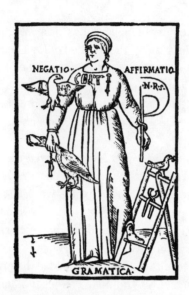

A memory figurine in the form of a personification of grammar. The inscriptions located around the figurine are memory cues for grammatical principles. Such figures are variations on the Method of Loci.

thus creating a memory palace for that information. Every liberal art was represented by a figure with a distinct persona. Grammar was portrayed as a stern old woman as we see here. Rhetoric, on the other hand, was more glamorous, depicted as a tall warrior princess carrying cues for various figures of speech. Other personifications provided images for logic, arithmetic, geometry, astronomy, and music. Ricci could well have studied such images, possibly customizing and elaborating them, to create memory palaces for key ideas in each subject.

By the end of his studies, Ricci would have had a sizable collection of memory palaces to take with him on his missionary adventures. His ability to use information from his education in future years was largely dependent on how well these memory aids functioned because there would be few Western books available to refresh his knowledge. His first stop was India, in 1578. He traveled with few personal possessions on a grueling six-month voyage by sail. In 1582 he left India for China, where he spent the rest of his life.

Ricci's first task there was to learn the language, and he applied his memory skills to the task. He studied Chinese ideographs and began to memorize them, almost certainly in a memory palace. By 1585 he was able to speak Chinese without an interpreter and read the language, albeit in a halting way. By 1594 he was fluent to the point where he could converse easily and compose letters and essays in Chinese that were well received by native speakers. In the process, he discovered that the Chinese were extremely interested in memory techniques. Following is his description of a party he attended in 1595 with the educated elite of Nanjing. The subject of memory strategies came up, and he offered to provide a demonstration.

> I told them they should write down a large number of Chinese letters in any manner they chose on a sheet of paper without there being any order among them, because after reading them only once, I would be able to say them all by heart in the same way and order in which they had been written. They did so, writing many letters without any order, all of which I, after reading them once, was able to repeat by memory in the manner in which they were written; such that they were all astonished, it seeming to them a great matter. And I, in order to increase their wonder, began to recite them all by memory backward in the same manner, beginning with the very last until reaching the first. By which they all became utterly astounded and as if beside themselves. And at once they began to beg me to consent to teach them this divine rule by which such a memory was made.

Here we see a master mnemonist at work. Spence, Ricci's biographer, believes that hundreds of ideographs were involved in this demonstration. If you experiment with memory palaces, you will discover they are not hard to use if you have plenty of time to create the necessary imagery. You will even find you can recall a list just as easily backward as forward. But using a palace as Ricci did, on the fly at the spur of the moment under pressure, is a totally different undertaking. His success shows the massive amount of practice he must have had with this technique.

The Chinese interest in memory gave Ricci an opening to build relationships with prominent people to increase his status and develop social contacts. One of these people was the governor of the province in which Nanjing is located, who was eager for his sons to do well on Chinese civil service exams. These difficult, high-stakes tests covered a staggering amount of material, and the results could significantly advance or hold back opportunities available to the young men who took them. Ricci offered to teach the governor's sons Western memory arts to prepare for the test. For that purpose, he wrote a small book in Chinese on memory palaces and presented copies of the book to the governor and his three sons. Unfortunately, his plan did not succeed, and the reason for its failure provides a valuable insight into the use of the Method of Loci.

It wasn't that the sons failed the exam—actually, they did well. They just did not find Ricci's memory techniques helpful and chose to study for the test in their own ways. In hindsight, this is not surprising. Although memory palaces are simple in concept, their application to complex material requires skill and experience. The three sons had to draw on only a written description of the technique to memorize a massive amount of difficult information without first practicing the system. Difficulties and discouragement were to be expected. A useful rule for anyone interested in using memory palaces is to start with modest projects and expect a learning curve.

Ricci's memory technique wasn't the only thing that interested the Chinese. They were hungry for Western knowledge of mathematics and science, as well as some aspects of philosophy. Ricci saw another way to open doors, and he began to prepare Chinese translations of these topics, translations that could be widely circulated to an influential readership. Ricci reasoned that if they liked these materials, they might become open to more religiously themed works.

In some cases, such as Euclid's *Elements of Geometry*, he worked from source books in Latin. But in others, Spence believes he wrote from memory. Spence found material in Ricci's Chinese books from exotic Western works that he almost certainly did not have access to in China—including passages from Aesop's fables and minor Greek philosophers and ancient Roman poets, excerpts from books whose importance could not have justified inclusion on Ricci's arduous travels. Spence found Ricci's translations faithful to the original sources. These were subjects Ricci had studied at the Jesuit College decades earlier, material he likely registered carefully in memory palaces he constructed at the time.

Long-Lasting Memories

If Spence is correct that many of Ricci's translations were from memory palaces created decades earlier, his memories were very durable indeed. Contemporary studies show that about thirty percent of the information learned in academic content courses—history, civics, psychology, science—is forgotten in the first year and that this number increases to as much as seventy percent after four years.

What explains the longevity of Ricci's memories? Two features of memory palaces may have contributed. First, establishing a memory palace requires deep processing, organization, and visualization. The result would be strong initial learning, a contributor to long-lasting memories. Second, once they are established, memory palaces allow a person to rehearse their content easily without study materials like books or notes. Ricci could at any time mentally journey through his palaces, recalling each fact in turn. For him, the palaces were mental versions of flashcards. Ricci was a committed student, and if he rehearsed material now and then during his college years, those rehearsals could have led to the kind of strong long-lasting memories I referred to in Chapter 9 as the "permastore." These are memories for academic content that you learn so well through spaced retrieval practice that they last for decades, sometimes as long as fifty years. For example, if you take a sequence of courses in Spanish, each of your classes provides another opportunity for you to rehearse vocabulary and grammar, leading to long-lasting memory even if you never use the language after college. So too it might have been with Ricci's memory palaces.

Memory Arts in Decline

Although memory training was well established in Catholic universities of Ricci's era, forces were in play that led to its decline in the broader European culture. The invention of printing a century earlier meant that books were now plentiful, eliminating a motivation for memory training. Critics lambasted memory training as rote, irrelevant learning, criticisms brought on by pedantic teachers who used the methods to force students to memorize useless facts. Protestant reformers asserted that the use of imagery in memory techniques was an ungodly Catholic practice that would lead to idolatry. There were also new ideas in the air with the Age of Reason and the Scientific Revolution just beginning. All of this meant that for a growing number the Method of Loci, with its places and images, was either (1) no longer needed, (2) too pedantic and rigid, (3) too Catholic, (4) too old school, or (5) some combination. The end result was that the memory strategies Ricci practiced with such great skill were on a slide into obscurity, and they never recovered.

Memory Palaces in the Twenty-First Century

There is no question that memory palaces served a valuable purpose in earlier times, but do these ancient mnemonic devices have any relevance in today's world? It's a fact that there are few situations outside of memory competitions where the Method of Loci is regularly put to use these days. This is probably due to the effort and practice the technique requires as well as ambiguity about just where you might use it in modern times. I was initially motivated to try the Method of Loci out of curiosity to see how it worked, but I quickly learned that memory palaces are not only fascinating as a mnemonic strategy but of genuine practical utility. Here are several of my memory projects to illustrate possibilities and perhaps suggest an application in your life.

Lists

Any of the list-based memory applications of the last chapter—shopping lists, to-do lists, appointments—can be handled with a memory palace. A memory palace is my mnemonic of choice when the list is long, say more than ten items. The most valuable application for me is as an aid to learning student names.

A few days before a new class begins, I put the names of students enrolled in the course into a memory palace I reserve just for this purpose. Its locations follow a route down a busy street and into a shopping mall. I know the area well, and I can easily travel it in my imagination. A typical class requires about thirty locations, although the route has accommodated as many as seventy. They are organized in sets of ten to aid in rehearsing them. Using the class list, I create a memory cue for each name at a specific spot. For example, if the name is "Elliot Beck" and the next location is a table at the Panda restaurant, I use the name-learning techniques of Chapter 7 to create an image at that spot to suggest Elliot's name. I might picture the politician "Eliot Spitzer" sporting a birdlike *beak* sitting at the table. Next I move to "Gretchen Burns" and create a memory image for her name in a specific chair at the Tiger Paws Nail Salon, the next location on my route. I rehearse the memory palace until I know the class list well—literally forwards and backwards. On the first day of class, when I meet each student, I associate a face with a name I already know, and that reduces my workload significantly. Immediately after class I go back through the memory palace. As I get to each name, I work on recalling the face that went with it to practice the connection. By the second week, I usually have learned peoples' names, and I no longer need the memory palace. I will slowly forget which names are where in the palace over the next few months, and I won't use the palace again until the next class.

A Personal Organizer

Andrew Card's impressive application of a memory palace to manage the White House was especially interesting to me because the content he remembered was constantly changing as new items were added and old ones became passé. I decided to experiment with a similar system just to see how it worked. That was almost a decade ago, and I continue to find it useful. It has replaced appointment calendars, memo pads, and sticky notes for managing details of my daily life.

This memory palace is located in my garage. It consists of a series of sites, like Card's kitchen stove with its four burners, each site with several locations for memory images. The first site in my palace is a shelf on the far wall of my garage next to the door. I imagine four objects on the shelf—a steel wedge for splitting wood, a garden digging tool, a box of plant food, and a hose nozzle—each is a possible location for a memory image. The objects are spaced evenly on the shelf and well illuminated. It's important to note that this shelf is in my imagination. The real shelf is not as orderly, and objects come and go from it. But the shelf in my memory palace will always be as it is. I remember miscellaneous tasks and appointments by associating a memory cue with one of the locations. For example, I need to renew my membership in a professional association, so I have an image of the steel wedge deeply driven into the group's logo, splitting it in two. The garden tool is associated with the next meeting of an advisory committee I serve on, and the plant food box has a big bite out of it to remind me of my next dental check-up. If I needed, I could create a memory aid for the date and time of the appointment, but it won't be necessary. I review the memory palace often, and when I get to the box, I refresh my memory of the appointment—May 7 at 9:00 A.M.

The next site is another shelf farther down the wall of the garage. It holds other objects that define locations for memory images. Today there are cues for a home repair I've been putting off, a broken drill bit I should replace and backup printer ink I need. When I take care of one of these tasks, it will be quickly forgotten, and the location will become available for a new item.

Ten additional sites follow, located in cabinets, in a tool box, in drawers, and on a workbench. Each site contains objects that serve as locations I associate with reminders relevant to a specific area of my life—a site for a community group I'm active in, one for my memory class, sites for hobbies and interests, one for family, another for friends, a site for health, and a place for this book project. I visit the memory palace almost every weekday morning. It is a peaceful time for me as I mentally go to each site to find what is stored there. When I'm finished, I have a plan for the day.

Remembering Facts

A traditional use for a memory palace is to hold static information such as the facts Ricci retained from his college days. I am a private pilot, and I have a memory palace devoted to aviation facts. It is constructed in my imagination around the plane I fly. I picture a domed structure on the left wing, and within it I have set up memory locations in three separate clusters. Each location contains images to cue facts about airspace rules and practices. In front of the plane, parked next to the propeller, is another imaginary memory area in the form of a large black FAA Suburban. Locations on the vehicle are associated with cues for various regulations. Protocols for different flight situations are represented by memory cues in an imaginary hangar on the right wing. Weather facts are on the tail surfaces. I use this memory palace primarily in the spring, at the beginning of my flying season, to rehearse and refresh key facts so that they'll easily come to mind if I need them.

In constructing a memory palace for facts, the suggestions presented in Chapter 9 are useful. The first step is to organize the material and segment it into bite-sized facts. Next is finding a cue for each that can be visually linked to a location in the memory palace. Once all the cues have been associated with specific locations, the facts can be rehearsed by mentally traveling through the palace.

The steps for remembering factual material are summarized in the Henry mnemonic from Chapter 9, shown again on the facing page. Henry's stop sign cues the process: Segment—Cue/Rehearse—Review. The Henry limerick, cued by the "H," emphasizes the importance of spaced rehearsal, and the dumbbell provides a cue for the Rule of Five. The "DD" stands for "desirable difficulty," a reminder that rehearsal will be most beneficial

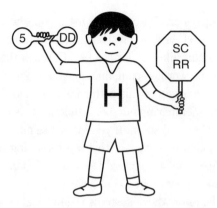

Henry, a mnemonic for ways to remember facts from Chapter 9. These same techniques can be applied to establishing facts in memory palaces.

when it requires some effort to recall the facts. A memory palace takes this approach for remembering facts to the next level.

Remembering a Deck of Cards

There is something about remembering the order of a deck of playing cards that appeals to people interested in the memory arts, and that includes me. It is one of the standard events at memory competitions, where the winners show astounding skill. The current world record for memorizing a single deck of fifty-two cards is twenty-one seconds. Former world champion Dominic O'Brien once memorized fifty-four decks of cards (2,808 total) in a single effort. These card-memory feats are done with memory palaces.

My ambitions are far more modest. For me, it's about a recreational challenge, not competition, and speed in memorizing is not a priority. I keep a deck of cards on my desk, and every now and then the deck catches my eye. I shuffle the cards and give it a go. When I remember them all, life is good.

The first requirement is to have a way to encode cards so that they can be placed in a memory palace. Card values, like "two of clubs" or "three of diamonds," are too bland to be remembered easily, so mnemonists associate them with concrete objects. My approach is similar to one described by Harry Lorayne and others. In it, a "two of clubs" becomes "coin" and a "three of diamonds" becomes "dame." Both are words that can be visualized in a memory palace. The complete list of code words is in the table below, and if you look closely, you'll see the pattern. Each code word begins with the letter of a suit, like "c" for "clubs." Cards of the same value have similar sounding code words—coin, dune, hen, and sun code the value "2" in the four suits. The origin of this pattern is the major system, described in Chapter 10, for remembering numbers. In it, a "2" is represented by "n," "3" by "m," "4" by "r," and so on. If you know the major system, this card code is particularly easy to learn, and that was its selling point for me. Memory competitors like Joshua Foer and Dominic O'Brien use more complex coding systems that allow them to put several cards at the same memory palace location. The effort these systems require makes sense when speed is the top priority. Even the less demanding system I use requires plenty

Concrete Words Used to Remember Specific Cards

| | Suit | | | |
	Clubs	Diamonds	Hearts	Spades
Ace	Cot	Date	Hat	Suit
2	Coin	Dune	Hen	Sun
3	Comb	Dame	Ham	Sum
4	Car	Door	Hare	Seer
5	Coal	Doll	Hail	Sail
6	Cage	Dash	Hash	Sash
7	Cake	Dock	Hog	Sock
8	Cave	Dove	Hoof	Safe
9	Cop	Dab	Hoop	Soap
10	Case	Dose	Hose	Suds
J	Club	Diamond	Heart	Spade
Q	Cream	Dream	Queen	Steam
K	King	Drink	Hinge	Sing

of practice with the code words to be facile with them, and this is essential before moving on to remembering cards. (If you decide to experiment with card memory, try starting out with one suit, say clubs, and get proficient in remembering the order of this group as a first step.)

The memory palace needs fifty-two locations. Mine begins in my home and continues around my neighborhood; it is organized in sets of 10. To remember the cards, I create an image linking the code word for each card to a location in the memory palace. So, if the current card is the four of hearts ("hare") and the current location is the mailbox on my neighbor's house, I imagine a rabbit with long ears and a woeful expression stuffed into the mailbox. The suggestions in Chapter 4 for memory images are helpful here. I make the images as distinctive and unique as I can manage and try to get them to interact with the locations in some way. Once I finish the cards, I come to my Moment of Truth when I recall them by going back through the palace.

A Final Thought

A memory palace makes use of two different features of our sophisticated visual system. One is the ability to remember locations so we can find our way in the environment. The other is the ability to remember the objects we encounter. These two features, memory for location and memory for objects, fulfill the two essential requirements of a list mnemonic: they organize material, and they provide encoding assistance to remember individual items. Together they make the Method of Loci the most powerful mnemonic system ever devised for retaining disconnected information that can be given a visual representation. Its most obvious use, of course, is to remember a list. But an application sometimes overlooked is using it to permit easy rehearsal of important information. Here the memory palace is used like flashcards to make memory strong enough that it can be recalled whenever it is needed without the palace.

In the Memory Lab:
A Memory Palace for This Book

This is the last installment of the Memory Lab, and in it I invite you to create a memory palace to help you recall a key point from each of the preceding chapters. Think of this as an approximation of the kinds of memory palaces Matteo Ricci used to remember college subjects.

The first step is to establish the locations in the palace. Select them on a fixed route you can physically travel such as around your home or in your neighborhood. For example, the route might be kitchen table → stove top → kitchen sink → bathroom tub → computer station → book shelf. You need thirteen locations. Mentally run over the route until you have it down.

The thirteen images you will place at these sites are shown on pages 218–220; there is one from each chapter, and they cue major ideas and memory strategies of the book. Before you begin to locate them in the memory palace, I suggest you prepare a written summary of the facts you want each image to cue. You can use it later to check your memory.

Now place the thirteen cues at the thirteen sites by imagining them interacting with these places. Rehearse the palace by moving through it, recalling each image and associated facts. One advantage of a memory palace is that you can rehearse anywhere, even in bed when you are slow getting to sleep. In fact, medieval monks believed that being in bed at night was one of the best settings for memory work because there are few distractions. Wherever you carry them out, spaced retrievals are essential if, like Matteo Ricci, you want to retain the information over time.

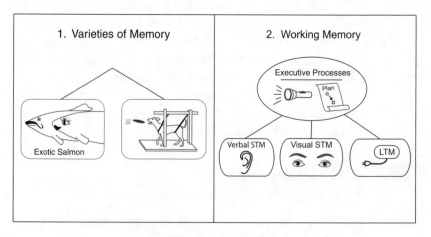

Memory images from Chapters 1–2.

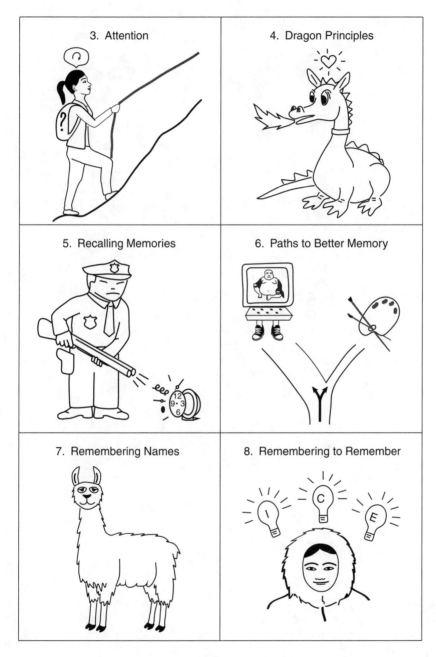

Memory images from Chapters 3–8.

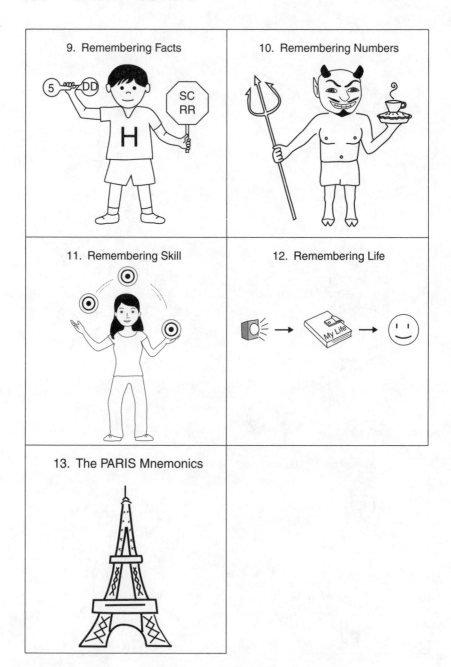

Memory images from Chapters 9–13.

15

Mindsets and Memory

Suppose you meet a nice couple at the dog park while you're watching your pet romp around. You chat, and later, as you are leaving, you bid them good-bye, calling each by name. This is a memory success, and you deserve to feel good about it as you and your dog head back to the car.

It's human nature to have an opinion about why you succeeded in remembering their names that day. Perhaps it was because your natural memory ability is especially good. Or maybe your success was due to the effort you put into remembering the names and the memory strategy you used. The difference between chalking up a success (or failure) to natural ability or to personal effort may seem like a trivial distinction. But it is not. The way you interpret memory outcomes can influence your attitude about your memory—how you think it functions and what it would take to improve it. That attitude can even affect what you try to remember.

Carol Dweck, a researcher at Stanford University, calls these two different attitudes "mindsets." With a fixed mindset you see your performance as the result of a relatively unchangeable ability like natural memory. A growth mindset is a belief that outcomes reflect your effort and technique, that improvement is possible if you work at it. To see these two mindsets at work, consider a study by Dweck and Claudia Mueller.

The two psychologists asked fifth-grade children to solve reasoning problems like the one on the next page. There were three separate work sessions. After the first session, each child was told he or she had done really well. Along with the good news, some children were praised for their natural ability: "You must be smart at these problems." Other children were praised for their effort: "You must have worked hard at these problems." Mueller and Dweck believed that these different forms of praise would encourage the children to adopt either a fixed or a growth mindset

Which answer completes the pattern?

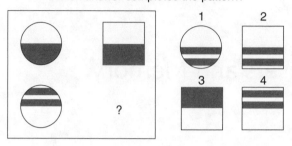

A reasoning problem similar to those given to fifth-grade children in the Mueller and Dweck study.

for evaluating their success, and the purpose of the study was to see if there were delayed consequences from the mindsets. The researchers suspected there could well be, especially if the children encountered a situation where they didn't succeed. After all, if doing well means you're smart, what does it mean when you fail? On the other hand, if doing well comes from working hard, failure has different implications.

To explore this issue, the researchers gave the children a dose of failure in the second work session, presenting them with a new set of problems much harder than the first. After the children finished, they were told that they had done a lot worse on the second set. Now the stage was set for the third session, when they were given problems similar to the easier ones they had first worked on. How would they rebound from failure? Would the kind of praise they received make a difference? The graph on page 223 compares the number of problems children solved in the first and third sessions. Those who had been praised for effort actually improved their performance, while those praised for ability showed a drop. What was going on?

Mueller and Dweck believe that the different mindsets gave failure different meanings for the two groups of children. When those who had been praised for being smart subsequently experienced failure, they were inclined to see it as a lack of ability, which made them less motivated to work on additional problems. The children who had been told they succeeded because they worked hard were likely to interpret the failure as a lack of effort, which led them to be more motivated in the third session.

The children also differed in the kinds of challenges they were willing to undertake in the future. Right after that first successful session, they

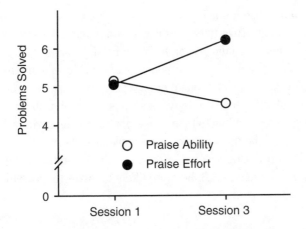

Performance on reasoning problems before and after a session where children experienced disappointing outcomes.

were asked what other kinds of reasoning problems they might like to work on. Most of those who had been praised for being smart (sixty-seven percent) chose options like "problems that aren't too hard so I won't get many wrong." They wanted to avoid failure, and they were drawn to safe choices involving easy problems. The children who had been praised for effort overwhelmingly (ninety-two percent) chose the option "problems I'd learn a lot from even if I won't look so smart." For these children, failure was much less negative, and they were attracted to challenging problems that offered a chance to learn better strategies.

There is now a large body of research on the importance of mindsets. A recent review summarized eighty-five studies and concluded that "mindsets matter." Whether people view ability as a skill that can be improved or a fixed entity influences many areas of human performance, including school achievement, success in sports, corporate leadership, dieting, and the dynamics of romantic relationships. Those with a growth mindset were more open to new learning; they were more resilient after failure, and they were more willing to take on challenges.

This insight is relevant to the practitioner of the memory arts. When you recall the movies nominated for this year's Academy Awards, and your friend says "You have a good memory," it's tempting to give credit to your natural memory. In fact, that's what your friend meant by the compliment. While this is flattering and empowering at the time, it is problematic in the long run because it doesn't prepare you to deal well with memory failures, which you are sure to experience at some point. This can limit your memory skill because failures can be more helpful than successes when it comes to improving memory—provided you are able to learn from them. Having the right mindset about memory outcomes, one that emphasizes growth through effort and strategy, sets the stage for improvement. It will also make you more willing to take on memory challenges where failure is a possibility—learning the names of new people in a group, retaining a phone number without writing it down, or making a presentation without notes. With a growth mindset, you'll be more likely to give situations like these a try and learn from them.

Mindsets and Stereotypes

A growth mindset is particularly beneficial to the elderly, who are bombarded with the widespread stereotype that advancing age leads to biologically driven cognitive decline and associated memory problems. Many older people embrace this notion, and we see evidence of it when someone forgets the name of a book he read last week or the dry cleaning she intended to pick up. Chagrined, they say "oops, a senior moment." The comment is understandable. Most elderly are aware that their memory is not as sharp as it once was, and the "senior moment" comment reflects this personal experience as well as societal stereotypes about aging. But in truth the actual reason for the memory slip will never be known—maybe it was age-related and maybe it wasn't. It is a fact that people of all ages forget. Calling this particular slip a "senior moment" will not be helpful if they're interested in improving their memory. To see why, think about what that expression means. It implies that the memory slip was a consequence of age and therefore is a permanent, fixed condition that will produce more memory errors in the future. Although it was a flip comment, it can undermine attempts to improve memory and even become a self-fulfilling prophecy—once this stereotype is taken to heart, expectations drop and the stage is set for lower memory performance regardless of any age-related factors that may or may not be operating.

Stereotype effects can be dramatic, as shown in a clever study of people between the ages of sixty and seventy conducted by Catherine Haslam and her colleagues at the University of Exeter. The participants were told that the purpose of the study was to investigate the way people of different ages performed on cognitive tests, and among the materials they were given was a magazine article about the association between aging and memory decline. Next came the ingenious twist in the experiment. Half the group was told that the study was made up of people between forty and seventy—this put them at the "old" end of the continuum. The other half was told that the study involved people between sixty and ninety, which put them at the "young" end. All the participants took a memory test—reading stories and then recalling them either immediately or after a thirty-minute delay. The results are shown in the bar graph below. Those who saw themselves as old conformed to the stereotype with poor memory performance. As you look at the figure, keep in mind that the only age difference between the two groups was in their minds.

Researchers have studied the impact of stereotypes on cognitive performance extensively, and the effects are well documented. The process begins when something in a situation triggers the stereotype, like the magazine article in the Haslam study. With the stereotype activated, those who thought of themselves as old tended to expect that they would do poorly on the coming memory test, and as a result they didn't try to the same extent as people who saw themselves as young.

Stereotype effects can have devastating consequences. Haslam and her colleagues found that activating an age stereotype can artificially lower

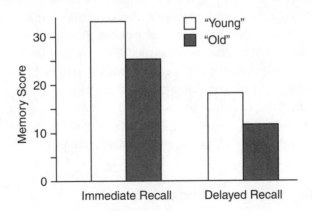

A comparison of memory test scores for senior citizens who thought they were either the youngest members of the group being tested ('young") or the oldest members of the group ("old").

some seniors' test scores on a screening exam to the point where they meet the diagnostic criteria for dementia, a diagnosis that is bad news indeed for the individual who receives it. For many elderly, dementia tops cancer as their most feared health affliction. And the diagnosis brings with it a new and even more pejorative stereotype.

The good news is that not everyone succumbs to stereotypes. Those most likely to accept them are people with fixed mindsets about abilities, and if they are in a vulnerable group like the elderly, they are more likely to apply the stereotype to themselves. When people are encouraged to adopt a growth mindset, they become less susceptible to stereotypes.

Researchers Jason Plaks and Allison Chasteen, working with a group of senior citizens in their seventies, investigated whether a change in mindset could have an immediate effect on memory. They gave some materials advocating a growth mindset and others materials supporting a fixed mindset. Next, all were given a memory test. Those who read material supporting a growth perspective outperformed the fixed mindset group by fifteen percent, a memory difference large enough that it could well be noticeable in daily life.

The elderly are not the only people who can derive special benefit from a growth mindset. Adopting this attitude can help anyone who has low expectations about their memory ability. This could be someone who has been diagnosed with a learning disability, or attention-deficit/hyperactivity disorder, or mild cognitive impairment, or a traumatic brain injury. Low expectations can also be a carryover from past performance problems, such as academic failures. Any one of these situations can create a nagging belief that you have a cognitive deficiency that includes a bad memory. When this belief is coupled with a fixed mindset that the cognitive abilities can't be improved, low expectations and weak motivation become locked in, creating an additional handicap that will further degrade performance. But a person's limitations can never be known with certainty. Adopting a growth mindset that says effort and strategy can improve performance will allow a person to move forward to the maximum extent possible.

Fostering a Growth Mindset

We pick up mindsets from the world around us—parents, peers, teachers, celebrities, and the media. They become our assumptions about how abilities come about and what can be done to improve them. We can have different mindsets for different abilities: for example, we might believe that athletic ability is fixed but that music ability comes about through practice, or vice versa. We can even hold both mindsets about the same ability, believing, for example, that although natural memory ability is fixed, memory skill can be improved with effort and strategy. These mindsets are not carved in stone. The studies reviewed in this chapter illustrate that mindsets can be changed by interventions such as the type of praise a teacher gives or the educational material people read.

A practitioner of the memory arts is in a good position to cultivate a growth mindset about memory because the techniques are based on learned skills and practice. But one more ingredient is necessary, and it has to do with the mnemonist's goals. Carol Dweck has identified two different forms achievement goals can take, and only one of them fully supports growth.

The one she recommends is called a "mastery goal," which focuses on developing and maintaining competence. Mastery goals are about taking on challenges and meeting them, and they accommodate failures as part of the process. Improvement is the name of the game. Dweck contrasts mastery goals with "performance goals," in which you seek praise for your successes and try to avoid the negative reactions that can result from failure. With performance goals the need to prevent failure becomes more important than the need to stretch and develop. When these goals dominate, progress in memory skill can be slowed or even derailed.

I believe that the best way to set the stage for continued progress is to deliberately interpret successes and disappointments as reflections of effort and strategy. Work on mastery goals, aim for small improvements, and find satisfaction in the process.

A Final Thought

A discussion of the growth mindset is an appropriate way to end this book. As we have seen in the previous chapters, there is abundant knowledge available about how to improve memory skill. Revolutionary advances in the scientific understanding of memory offer a better foundation than ever before for memory strategies that address the challenges of daily life—names and faces, numbers and facts, skills and intentions, even the events of your own life. To take advantage of real opportunities for memory development, all you need to add is a growth mindset and a commitment to improving your skill.

It's ironic that so many possibilities for improving memory have become available at the same time all manner of electronic devices have appeared to manage the information in our lives, relieving us of the need to be responsible for retaining it ourselves. When it comes to storing and accessing information, it could be argued that the need for traditional memory arts is on the wane. Given a smartphone and an Internet connection, you can meet many of the memory challenges I've addressed in this book. But people who are drawn to the memory arts—and I hope this book has helped make you one of them—are not motivated solely by managing information, just as a person who chooses to walk rather than drive is motivated by more than getting from point A to point B. Walking or biking offers opportunities for self-reliance, healthy exercise, and personal satisfaction. So it is with memory. Memory strategies and techniques are a complement, or even an antidote, to electronic devices, which have become so useful and seductive that they foster alarming levels of dependency.

I hope you'll take on the challenge of strengthening your memory in some area of your life, whether it be remembering names or studying more effectively or learning a new skill. And for readers who have a deeper commitment to mnemonic techniques, those who only grudgingly resort to sticky notes and the like, I offer this:

Every Day
Find a Way
To Put in Play
The Memory Arts

Notes

Introduction

Page 1

Here is Dan Rookwood: Rookwood, D. (2011, August 24). Technology overload. Retrieved May 12, 2014, from *www.gq.com.au/life/editors+pick/technology+overload,13897.*

Page 2

A survey of 3,000 Britons: Quinn, B. (2007, July 13). Mobile phones "dumbing down brain power." Retrieved May 12, 2014, from *www.telegraph.co.uk/news/uknews/1557293/Mobile-phones-dumbing-down-brain-power.html.*

Page 3

consider the story of Scott Hagwood: Hagwood, S. (2007). *Memory power: You can develop a great memory—America's Grand Master shows you how.* New York: Free Press.

Page 3

Hagwood bought a book: Buzan, T. (1991). *Use your perfect memory: Dramatic new techniques for improving your memory* (3rd ed.). New York: Plume.

Chapter 1

Page 9

H. M.'s epilepsy resulted from: Two books were my sources for details about H. M. Corkin, S. (2013). *Permanent present tense: The unforgettable life of the amnesic patient, H. M.* New York: Basic Books; and Hilts, P. J. (1996). *Memory's ghost: The nature of memory and the strange tale of Mr. M.* New York: Touchstone.

Page 10
Scoville was undeterred: In 1974, Scoville called the operation "a tragic mistake" (Corkin, 2013, p. 47).

Page 10
As Milner told a reporter: Hilts (1996, p. 110).

Page 10
"This patient's memory defect": Scoville, W. B., & Milner, B. (1957). Loss of recent memory after bilateral hippocampal lesions. *Journal of Neurology, Neurosurgery and Psychiatry, 20*, 14.

Page 11
Milner's ongoing work: This research was reported in 1962 in an obscure paper that is summarized in Milner, B., Squire, L., & Kandel, E. (1998). Cognitive neuroscience and the study of memory. *Neuron, 20*, 445–468. The figure on page 12 was derived from the data presented in their Figure 2.

Page 12
a different picture emerged: Squire, L. R. (2004). Memory systems of the brain: A brief history and current perspective. *Neurobiology of Learning and Memory, 82*(3), 171–177.

Page 13
Tulving proposed: Tulving, E. (2002). Episodic memory: From mind to brain. *Annual Review of Psychology, 53*(1), 1–25.

Page 14
Children develop the ability to time travel: Russell, J., Alexis, D., & Clayton, N. (2010). Episodic future thinking in 3- to 5-year-old children: The ability to think of what will be needed from a different point of view. *Cognition, 114*(1), 56–71.

Page 14
Older adults who have trouble remembering: Addis, D. R., Wong, A. T., & Schacter, D. L. (2008). Age-related changes in the episodic simulation of future events. *Psychological Science, 19*(1), 33–41.

Page 14
Tulving believes that this kind: Tulving, E. (2005). Episodic memory and autonoesis: Uniquely human? In H. S. Terrace & J. Metcalfe (Eds.), *The missing link in cognition: Origins of self-reflective consciousness* (pp. 3–56). New York: Oxford University Press.

Page 14

Semantic memory is thought to start: Diekelmann, S., & Born, J. (2010). The memory function of sleep. *Nature Reviews Neuroscience, 11*(2), 114–126.

Page 15

Such memories are called "implicit": The distinction between explicit and implicit memory is also referred to as a distinction between "declarative" and "nondeclarative" memory. The terminology is used interchangeably in research reports.

Page 16

Ronald Reagan's struggle: Altman, L. (1997, October 5). Reagan's twilight— A special report: A president fades into a world apart. *New York Times.* Retrieved from *www.nytimes.com/1997/10/05/us/reagan-s-twilight-a-special-report-a-president-fades-into-a-world-apart.html*

Page 17

expert radiologists: Myles-Worsley, M., Johnston, W. A., & Simons, M. A. (1988). The influence of expertise on X-ray image processing. *Journal of Experimental Psychology: Learning, Memory, and Cognition, 14*(3), 553–557.

Page 17

experienced computer programmers: Davies, S. P. (1991). The role of notation and knowledge representation in the determination of programming strategy: A framework for integrating models of programming behavior. *Cognitive Science, 15*(4), 547–572.

Page 17

the best-known psychology experiment: The drawing is from Yerkes, R. M., & Morgulis, S. (1909). The method of Pawlow in animal psychology. *Psychological Bulletin, 6*(8), 257–273.

Page 17

He described the curious case: Claparède, E. (1911/1995). Recognition and selfhood (Ann-Marie Bonnel, Trans.). *Consciousness and Cognition, 4,* 371–378.

Page 20

Cicero spoke for many ancients: Cicero, *De orotore,* II, lxxxvii, 357.

Page 21

the "substitute word technique": This terminology is from Lorayne, H., & Lucas, J. (1974). *The memory book.* Briarcliff Manor, NY: Stein and Day. Lorayne promoted the technique to remember abstract words, people's last names, and foreign vocabulary. When used to remember foreign vocabulary words, the technique has been called the "keyword mnemonic" by psychologists and has been studied extensively. This research is reviewed by Worthen, J. B., & Hunt, R. R. (2010). *Mnemonology: Mnemonics for the 21st century.* New York: Psychology Press. Also see Desrochers, A., & Begg, I. (1987). A theoretical account of encoding and retrieval processes in the use of imagery-based mnemonic techniques: The special case of the keyword method. In M. McDaniel & M. Pressley (Eds.), *Imagery and related mnemonic processes: Theories, individual differences, and applications* (pp. 56–77). New York: Springer-Verlag.

Page 23

about as much memory enhancement: McKelvie, S. J. (1995). The VVIQ as a psychometric test of individual differences in visual imagery vividness: A critical quantitative review and plea for direction. *Journal of Mental Imagery, 19*(3–4), 1–106.

Chapter 2

Page 24

Short-Order Cook: Daniels, J. (1985). *Places/Everyone.* Madison: University of Wisconsin Press. Copyright 1985 by the Board of Regents of the University of Wisconsin System. Reprinted by permission of The University of Wisconsin Press.

Page 27

the work of influential British researcher Alan Baddeley: Baddeley, A. (2007). *Working memory, thought, and action.* New York: Oxford University Press.

Page 28

the seat of consciousness: Baddeley (2007, pp. 314–316).

Page 28

was prepared from one such source: The averages for ages eighteen through eighty-seven are from Table B.6 in Wechsler, D. (1997). *WAIS-III administration and scoring manual* (3rd ed.). San Antonio, TX: Psychological Corp. The averages for ages six, eight, ten, twelve, and fourteen are from Table B.7 in Wechsler, D. (2003). *WISC-IV administration and scoring manual* (4th ed.). San Antonio, TX: Psychological Corp. The ninetieth and tenth percentiles are estimates calculated as plus and minus 1.28 times the standard deviation values given in the tables.

Page 29

only a moderate decline over the lifespan: Alloway, T. P., & Alloway, R. G. (2013). Working memory across the lifespan: A cross-sectional approach. *Journal of Cognitive Psychology, 25*(1), 84–93. Larger age effects are found for visuospatial working memory than verbal working memory. See Murre, J. M. J., Janssen, S. M. J., Rouw, R., & Meeter, M. (2013). The rise and fall of immediate and delayed memory for verbal and visuospatial information from late childhood to late adulthood. *Acta Psychologica, 142*(1), 96–107.

Page 30

what bedevils older people: Darowski, E. S., Helder, E., Zacks, R. T., Hasher, L., & Hambrick, D. Z. (2008). Age-related differences in cognition: The role of distraction control. *Neuropsychology, 22*(5), 638–644.

Page 30

reading comprehension can be predicted: Daneman, M., & Carpenter, P. A. (1980). Individual differences in working memory and reading. *Journal of Verbal Learning and Verbal Behavior, 19*(4), 450–466.

Page 30

In tests of reasoning ability: Oberauer, K., Süß, H.-M., Wilhelm, O., & Sander, N. (2008). Individual differences in working memory capacity and reasoning ability. In A. R. A. Conway, C. Jarrold, M. J. Kane, & J. N. Towse (Eds.), *Variation in working memory* (pp. 49–75). New York: Oxford University Press.

Page 30

Students mastering a computer language: Shute, V. J. (1991). Who is likely to acquire programming skills? *Journal of Educational Computing Research, 7*(1), 1–24.

Page 30

In a study of airplane pilots: Sohn, Y. W., & Doane, S. M. (2004). Memory processes of flight situation awareness: Interactive roles of working memory capacity, long-term working memory, and expertise. *Human Factors, 46*(3), 461–475.

Page 30

The connection to working memory: Conway, A. R. A., Cowan, N., Bunting, M. F., Therriault, D. J., & Minkoff, S. R. B. (2002). A latent variable analysis of working memory capacity, short-term memory capacity, processing speed, and general fluid intelligence. *Intelligence, 30*(2), 163–184.

Page 32

"We're back to the action": Hambrick, D. Z., & Engle, R. W. (2002). Effects of domain knowledge, working memory capacity, and age on cognitive performance: An investigation of the knowledge-is-power hypothesis. *Cognitive Psychology, 44*(4), 339–387.

Page 33

their findings are shown in the bar graph: From Table 9 in Hambrick & Engle (2002).

Page 34

In a definitive analysis: Cowan, N. (2000). The magical number 4 in short-term memory: A reconsideration of mental storage capacity. *Behavioral and Brain Sciences, 24*, 87–114. Also see Cowan, N. (2010). The magical mystery four: How is working memory capacity limited, and why? *Current Directions in Psychological Science, 19*(1), 51–57.

Page 34

to some extent may be inherited: Ando, J., Ono, Y., & Wright, M. J. (2001). Genetic structure of spatial and verbal working memory. *Behavior Genetics, 31*(6), 615–624.

Page 36

The Picture Superiority Effect: Classic studies are described by Paivio, A. (1971). *Imagery and verbal processes.* New York: Holt, Rinehart & Winston. A summary of theories to explain the picture superiority effect appears in McBride, D. M., & Dosher, B. A. (2002). A comparison of conscious and automatic memory processes for picture and word stimuli: A process dissociation analysis. *Consciousness and Cognition, 11*(3), 423–460.

Page 36

Researchers estimate: Van Essen, D. C., Anderson, C. H., & Felleman, D. J. (1992). Information processing in the primate visual system: An integrated systems perspective. *Science, 255*(5043), 419–423.

Chapter 3

Page 38

On an August evening in 1967: The most complete account of Margetts's story is Shapreau, C. (2006, February 12). Lost and found. And lost again? *Los Angeles Times.* Retrieved from *www.latimes.com/local/la-tm-violin7feb12-story.html#page=1.*

Page 40

"The secret of a good memory is attention": Edwards, T. (1891). *A dictionary of thoughts: Being a cyclopedia of laconic quotations from the best authors, both* *ancient and modern*, p. 342. New York: Cassell. Retrieved from *http://books. google.com/books*.

Page 41

One of their attention tests: A study that used the attention control test is Kane, M. J., Bleckley, M. K., Conway, A. R. A., & Engle, R. W. (2001). A controlled-attention view of working-memory capacity. *Journal of Experimental Psychology: General, 130*(2), 169–183.

Page 41

A large body of research supports: McCabe, D. P., Roediger, H. L., McDaniel, M. A., Balota, D. A., & Hambrick, D. Z. (2010). The relationship between working memory capacity and executive functioning: Evidence for a common executive attention construct. *Neuropsychology, 24*(2), 222–243.

Page 42

The two forms of attention evolved together: Allport, A. (1989). Visual attention. In M. I. Posner (Ed.), *Foundations of cognitive science* (pp. 631–663). Cambridge, MA: MIT Press.

Page 43

The third network is neurologically distinct: Buckner, R. L., Andrews-Hanna, J. R., & Schacter, D. L. (2008). The brain's default network: Anatomy, function, and relevance to disease. *Annals of the New York Academy of Sciences, 1124*, 1–38.

Page 44

Researcher Jonathan Smallwood calls this type: Smallwood, J., McSpadden, M., & Schooler, J. W. (2008). When attention matters: The curious incident of the wandering mind. *Memory and Cognition, 36*(6), 1144–1150.

Page 44

In one study, research participants were fitted: Reichle, E. D., Reineberg, A. E., & Schooler, J. W. (2010). Eye movements during mindless reading. *Psychological Science, 21*(9), 1300–1310.

Page 46

Researchers have found that restoring working memory: Clapp, W. C., Rubens, M. T., & Gazzaley, A. (2010). Mechanisms of working memory disruption by external interference. *Cerebral Cortex, 20*(4), 859–872.

Page 47

As the exam sits on his desk: A review of studies examining how worry, self-talk, and interfering thoughts affect test anxiety and performance is provided by Zeidner, M. (1998). *Test anxiety: The state of the art*, pp. 31–40. New York: Plenum Press.

Page 48
Athletes and coaches are well aware: Hatzigeorgiadis, A., Zourbanos, N., Galanis, E., & Theodorakis, Y. (2011). Self-talk and sports performance: A meta-analysis. *Perspectives on Psychological Science, 6*(4), 348–356.

Page 48
"just do it": Cousins, S. O., & Gillis, M. M. (2005). "Just do it . . . before you talk yourself out of it": The self-talk of adults thinking about physical activity. *Psychology of Sport and Exercise, 6*(3), 313–334.

Page 48
"Am I going to do this or not?": Senay, I., Albarracín, D., & Noguchi, K. (2010). Motivating goal-directed behavior through introspective self-talk: The role of the interrogative form of simple future tense. *Psychological Science, 21*(4), 499–504.

Page 48
help test-anxious students stay focused on the test: Zeidner (1998, pp. 373–377).

Page 48
which enhances motivation by activating: Kang, M. J., Hsu, M., Krajbich, I. M., Loewenstein, G., McClure, S. M., Wang, J. T., & Camerer, C. F. (2009). The wick in the candle of learning: Epistemic curiosity activates reward circuitry and enhances memory. *Psychological Science, 20*(8), 963–973.

Page 48
"When it is said that attention will not take a firm hold": Halleck, R. P. (1895). *Psychology and psychic culture*, p. 54. New York: American Book. Retrieved from *http://books.google.com/books*.

Page 49
"Flow is a subjective state": Csikszentmihalyi, M., Abuhamdeh, S., & Nakamura, J. (2005). Flow. In A. J. Elliot & C. S. Dweck (Eds.), *Handbook of competence and motivation* (pp. 598–608). New York: Guilford Press.

Chapter 4

Page 54
A retention intention sets the stage for good remembering: Specifying a plan in advance and committing to it is called an "implementation intention," a powerful cognitive strategy discussed in Chapter 8.

Page 55

In an important study: Craik, F. I. M., & Tulving, E. (1975). Depth of processing and the retention of words in episodic memory. *Journal of Experimental Psychology: General, 104*(3), 268–294. The figure on page 55 plots data from their Figure 3 for "yes" responses to "words presented twice."

Page 56

Deep processing even shows up in brain scans: Nyberg, L. (2002). Levels of processing: A view from functional brain imaging. *Memory, 10*(5–6), 345–348.

Page 57

One of the best ways to elaborate memory: Pressley, M., McDaniel, M. A., Turnure, J. E., Wood, E., & Ahmad, M. (1987). Generation and precision of elaboration: Effects on intentional and incidental learning. *Journal of Experimental Psychology: Learning, Memory, and Cognition, 13*(2), 291–300.

Page 58

Primal themes like survival: Nairne, J. S., & Pandeirada, J. N. S. (2008). Adaptive memory: Is survival processing special? *Journal of Memory and Language, 59*(3), 377–385.

Page 58

In one notable effort, Lionel Standing: Standing, L. (1973). Learning 10,000 pictures. *Quarterly Journal of Experimental Psychology, 25*(2), 207–222.

Page 58

Peter of Ravenna: Yates, F. A. (1966). *The art of memory,* p. 120. London: Pimlico.

Page 58

Francesco Panigarola: Spence, J. D. (1985). *The memory palace of Matteo Ricci,* p. 9. New York: Penguin Books.

Page 59

"Now nature herself teaches us": Appears in Yates (1966, p. 25).

Page 59

"Suppose someone must memorize": Appears in Carruthers, M., & Ziolkowski, J. M. (2003). *The medieval craft of memory: An anthology of texts and pictures,* pp. 209–210. Philadelphia: University of Pennsylvania Press.

Page 59

Modern research shows: The effectiveness of bizarre imagery is reported by McDaniel, M. A., & Einstein, G. O. (1986). Bizarre imagery as an effective memory aid: The importance of distinctiveness. *Journal of Experimental Psychology: Learning, Memory, and Cognition, 12*(1), 54–65. Benefits at longer retrieval intervals were found by O'Brien, E. J., & Wolford, C. R. (1982). Effect of delay in testing on retention of plausible versus bizarre mental images. *Journal of Experimental Psychology: Learning, Memory, and Cognition, 8*(2), 148–152.

Page 60

Colored images are five to ten percent: Wichmann, F. A., Sharpe, L. T., & Gegenfurtner, K. R. (2002). The contributions of color to recognition memory for natural scenes. *Journal of Experimental Psychology: Learning, Memory, and Cognition, 28*(3), 509–520.

Page 60

Movement has also been shown: Matthews, W. J., Benjamin, C., & Osborne, C. (2007). Memory for moving and static images. *Psychonomic Bulletin and Review, 14*(5), 989–993.

Page 61

Dominic O'Brien, a legendary memory competitor: O'Brien, D. (2000). *Learn to remember: Practical techniques and exercises to improve your memory,* p. 65. San Francisco: Chronicle Books.

Page 61

Harry Lorayne: Lorayne, H. (2007). *Ageless memory: Simple secrets for keeping your brain young,* p. 86. New York: Black Dog & Leventhal.

Page 61

Joshua Foer: Foer, J. (2011). *Moonwalking with Einstein: The art and science of remembering everything,* p. 3. New York: Penguin Press.

Page 62

Later, when he is trying to retrieve: Foer (2011, p. 183).

Page 63

one of the best established principles: Dempster, F. N. (1988). The spacing effect: A case study in the failure to apply the results of psychological research. *American Psychologist, 43*(8), 627–634.

Page 63

"Rule of Five": O'Brien (2000, p. 81).

Page 63

Other mnemonists offer similar spacing advice: Hagwood, S. (2007). *Memory power: You can develop a great memory—America's Grand Master shows you how,* p. 72. London: Free Press. Lorayne, H., & Lucas, J. (1974). *The memory book,* p. 32. Briarcliff Manor, NY: Stein & Day.

Page 64

In a now classic study: Bower, G. H., Clark, M. C., Lesgold, A. M., & Winzenz, D. (1969). Hierarchical retrieval schemes in recall of categorized word lists. *Journal of Verbal Learning and Verbal Behavior, 8*(3), 323–343.

Page 64

"What assists the memory most?": The memory teacher was Consultus Fortunatianus. His memory advice appears in Carruthers & Ziolkowski (2003, pp. 296–297).

Page 64

"a single glance of the mind's eye": Carruthers, M. (1998). *The craft of thought: Meditation, rhetoric, and the making of images, 400–1200*, p. 63. New York: Cambridge University Press.

Chapter 5

Page 69

"Having lived most of his life": Smith, S. M. (1988). Environmental context—dependent memory, p. 13. In G. M. Davies & D. M. Thomson (Eds.), *Memory in context: Context in memory.* Oxford, UK: John Wiley & Sons.

Page 70

Memory trainer Tony Buzan recommends: Buzan, T. (1991). *Use your perfect memory: Dramatic new techniques for improving your memory* (3rd ed.), pp. 161–162. New York: Plume.

Page 71

It has been shown to recover: Fisher, R. P., & Geiselman, R. E. (2010). The cognitive interview method of conducting police interviews: Eliciting extensive information and promoting therapeutic jurisprudence. *International Journal of Law and Psychiatry, 33*(5–6), 321–328.

Page 71

"Try to put yourself back": Fisher, R. P., & Geiselman, R. E. (1992). *Memory-enhancing techniques for investigative interviewing: The cognitive interview*, p. 100. Springfield, IL: Charles C Thomas.

Page 71

conducted an instructive experiment: Erdelyi, M. H., & Kleinbard, J. (1978). Has Ebbinghaus decayed with time? The growth of recall (hypermnesia) over days. *Journal of Experimental Psychology: Human Learning and Memory, 4*(4), 275–289. The figure on page 72 is based on their Figure 3.

Page 72

The strategy aids memory in two ways: Payne, D. G. (1987). Hypermnesia and reminiscence in recall: A historical and empirical review. *Psychological Bulletin, 101*(1), 5–27. Mulligan, N. W. (2006). Hypermnesia and total retrieval time. *Memory, 14*(4), 502–518.

Page 73

You will combine the gist and specifics: My presentation follows the fuzzy trace theory of Brainerd, C. J., & Reyna, V. F. (2005). *The science of false memory*, pp. 83–91. New York: Oxford University Press.

Page 74

"dumped in and tagged": Moscovitch, M. (2008). The hippocampus as a "stupid," domain-specific module: Implications for theories of recent and remote memory, and of imagination. *Canadian Journal of Experimental Psychology, 62*(1), 66.

Page 75

Researchers believe that memories briefly enter a malleable phase: Dudai, Y. (2012). The restless engram: Consolidations never end. *Annual Review of Neuroscience, 35*, 227–247.

Page 75

responses from a pair of identical twins: Sheen, M., Kemp, S., & Rubin, D. C. (2006). Disputes over memory ownership: What memories are disputed? *Genes, Brain and Behavior, 5*(Suppl. 1), 9–13.

Page 76

Most of the twin pairs: Sheen, M., Kemp, S., & Rubin, D. (2001). Twins dispute memory ownership: A new false memory phenomenon. *Memory and Cognition, 29*(6), 779–788.

Page 76

We can even mix up information: Loftus, E. F. (2005). Planting misinformation in the human mind: A 30-year investigation of the malleability of memory. *Learning and Memory, 12*(4), 361–366.

Page 76

Loftus began her study: Loftus, E. F., & Pickrell, J. E. (1995). The formation of false memories. *Psychiatric Annals, 25*(12), 720–725.

Page 77

Other researchers have replicated: Hyman, I. E., Husband, T. H., & Billings, F. J. (1995). False memories of childhood experiences. *Applied Cognitive Psy-*

chology, 9(3), 181–197. Porter, S., Yuille, J. C., & Lehman, D. R. (1999). The nature of real, implanted, and fabricated memories for emotional childhood events: Implications for the recovered memory debate. *Law and Human Behavior, 23*(5), 517–537.

Page 77

when they were debriefed: Loftus & Pickrell (1995, p. 723).

Page 77

memory confidence has been shown: Wells, G. L., Memon, A., & Penrod, S. D. (2006). Eyewitness evidence: Improving its probative value. *Psychological Science in the Public Interest, 7*(2), 45–75.

Page 77

two hundred cases in which DNA evidence: DNA exonerations are tracked by The Innocence Project. Retrieved June 15, 2014, from *www.innocenceproject. org.*

Page 77

there is no completely reliable way: Bernstein, D. M., & Loftus, E. F. (2009). How to tell if a particular memory is true or false. *Perspectives on Psychological Science, 4*(4), 370–374.

Chapter 6

Page 83

Memory, he wrote: Cicero, M. T. (1890). *Orations of Marcus Tullius Cicero,* p. 528. (C. D. Yonge, Trans.) (Vol. 4). London: Bell & Daldy. Retrieved from *http://books.google.com/books.*

Page 83

memory took two forms: Yates, F. A. (1966). *The art of memory.* London: Pimlico.

Page 84

"If I am asked what is the one great art of memory": Quintilian 11.2.40.

Page 84

William James . . . put the idea to the test: James, W. (1890). *The principles of psychology: Authorized edition, unabridged* (Vol. 1, pp. 667–668). New York: Dover Publications. Retrieved from *http://books.google.com/books.*

Page 84

Edward Thorndike, a leader in the early research: Thorndike, E. L. (1911).

The principles of teaching: Based on psychology, p. 241. New York: A. G. Seiler. Retrieved from *http://books.google.com/books*.

Page 85

published by Swedish researcher: Klingberg, T., Fernell, E., Olesen, P. J., Johnson, M., Gustafsson, P., Dahlström, K., et al. (2005). Computerized training of working memory in children with ADHD—A randomized, controlled trial. *Journal of the American Academy of Child and Adolescent Psychiatry, 44*(2), 177–186.

Page 85

all of whom show working memory problems: The connection between working memory and ADHD is reviewed by Alderson, R. M., Kasper, L. J., Hudec, K. L., & Patros, C. H. G. (2013). Attention-deficit/hyperactivity disorder (ADHD) and working memory in adults: A meta-analytic review. *Neuropsychology, 27*(3), 287–302. The role of working memory in beginning reading and mathematics education is examined by Gathercole, S., & Alloway, T. P. (2008). *Working memory and learning: A practical guide for teachers*. Los Angeles, CA: SAGE.

Page 86

The mood in the research community: Melby-Lervåg, M., & Hulme, C. (2013). Is working memory training effective? A meta-analytic review. *Developmental Psychology, 49*(2), 270–291. Rabipour, S., & Raz, A. (2012). Training the brain: Fact and fad in cognitive and behavioral remediation. *Brain and Cognition, 79*(2), 159–179. Shipstead, Z., Redick, T. S., & Engle, R. W. (2012). Is working memory training effective? *Psychological Bulletin, 138*(4), 628–654.

Page 87

The market for brain-fitness software: Jones, S. M. (2011, March 1). Retailer banks on brain fitness to expand stores. Retrieved June 16, 2014, from *http://articles.chicagotribune.com/2011-03-01/business/ct-biz-0302-marbles-20110301_1_brain-fitness-retailer-banks-sales-associates*.

Page 87

Jungle Memory spare no words: Retrieved June 15, 2014, from *http://junglememory.com/pages/how_it_works*.

Page 87

Mindsparke's pitch: Retrieved June 15, 2014, from *www.mindsparke.com/better_memory.php*.

Page 88

published in the prestigious British journal: Owen, A. M., Hampshire, A.,

Grahn, J. A., Stenton, R., Dajani, S., Burns, A. S., et al. (2010). Putting brain training to the test. *Nature, 465*(7299), 775–778.

Page 88
It has been described as: Kabat-Zinn, J. (1994). *Wherever you go, there you are,* pp. 3–9. New York: Hyperion.

Page 88
developed a widely adopted eight-week mindfulness training program: Kabat-Zinn, J. (1990). *Full catastrophe living?: Using the wisdom of your body and mind to face stress, pain, and illness.* New York: Bantam.

Page 89
Christian Jensen and his collaborators: Jensen, C. G., Vangkilde, S., Frokjaer, V., & Hasselbalch, S. G. (2012). Mindfulness training affects attention—Or is it attentional effort? *Journal of Experimental Psychology: General, 141*(1), 106–123.

Page 89
especially for attention: Chiesa, A., Calati, R., & Serretti, A. (2011). Does mindfulness training improve cognitive abilities? A systematic review of neuropsychological findings. *Clinical Psychology Review, 31*(3), 449–464.

Page 89
Memory also seems to profit: Chambers, R., Lo, B. C. Y., & Allen, N. B. (2008). The impact of intensive mindfulness training on attentional control, cognitive style, and affect. *Cognitive Therapy and Research, 32*(3), 303–322. Mrazek, M. D., Franklin, M. S., Phillips, D. T., Baird, B., & Schooler, J. W. (2013). Mindfulness training improves working memory capacity and GRE performance while reducing mind wandering. *Psychological Science, 24*(5), 776–781.

Page 89
ability to remember old personal memories: Heeren, A., Van Broeck, N., & Philippot, P. (2009). The effects of mindfulness on executive processes and autobiographical memory specificity. *Behaviour Research and Therapy, 47*(5), 403–409.

Page 90
In one large project: Laurin, D., Verreault, R., Lindsay, J., MacPherson, K., & Rockwood, K. (2001). Physical activity and risk of cognitive impairment and dementia in elderly persons. *Archives of Neurology, 58*(3), 498–504.

Page 90
Arthur Kramer and his associates: Kramer, A. F., Hahn, S., McAuley, E., Cohen, N. J., Banich, M. T., Harrison, C., et al. (2001). Exercise, aging, and

cognition: Healthy body, healthy mind? In W. A. Rogers & A. D. Fisk (Eds.), *Human factors interventions for the health care of older adults* (pp. 91–120). Mahwah, NJ: Lawrence Erlbaum.

Page 90

These results have been confirmed: Guiney, H., & Machado, L. (2013). Benefits of regular aerobic exercise for executive functioning in healthy populations. *Psychonomic Bulletin and Review, 20*(1), 73–86. Smith, P. J., Blumenthal, J. A., Hoffman, B. M., Cooper, H., Strauman, T. A., Welsh-Bohmer, K., et al. (2010). Aerobic exercise and neurocognitive performance: A meta-analytic review of randomized controlled trials. *Psychosomatic Medicine, 72*(3), 239–252. Voss, M. W., Nagamatsu, L. S., Liu-Ambrose, T., & Kramer, A. F. (2011). Exercise, brain, and cognition across the life span. *Journal of Applied Physiology, 111*(5), 1505–1513.

Page 91

show better academic achievement: Grissom, J. B. (2005). Physical fitness and academic achievement. *Journal of Exercise Physiology, 8*(1), 11–25.

Page 91

fit children have more brain volume: Chaddock, L., Pontifex, M. B., Hillman, C. H., & Kramer, A. F. (2011). A review of the relation of aerobic fitness and physical activity to brain structure and function in children. *Journal of the International Neuropsychological Society, 17*(6), 975–985.

Page 91

results suggest small improvements: Kamijo, K., Pontifex, M. B., O'Leary, K. C., Scudder, M. R., Wu, C., Castelli, D. M., et al. (2011). The effects of an afterschool physical activity program on working memory in preadolescent children. *Developmental Science, 14*(5), 1046–1058. Tomporowski, P. D., Lambourne, K., & Okumura, M. S. (2011). Physical activity interventions and children's mental function: An introduction and overview. *Preventive Medicine, 52*(Suppl.), S3–S9.

Page 91

twelve weeks of aerobic exercise: Pereira, A. C., Huddleston, D. E., Brickman, A. M., Sosunov, A. A., Hen, R., McKhann, G. M., et al. (2007). An in vivo correlate of exercise-induced neurogenesis in the adult dentate gyrus. *PNAS Proceedings of the National Academy of Sciences of the United States of America, 104*(13), 5638–5643.

Page 91

follow government guidelines: Retrieved June 15, 2014, from *www.cdc.gov/physicalactivity/everyone/guidelines/adults.html.*

Page 92

based on average gains found in available research: Computer training improvements were taken from the meta-analysis of Melby-Lervåg & Hulme (2013). The working memory gain plotted at point *a* is the percentile equivalent of Cohen's $d = 0.65$, the mean of the verbal ($d = 0.79$) and visuospatial values ($d = 0.52$) given in the paper. The transfer effect size plotted as point *c* corresponds to Cohen's $d = 0.16$, the average of verbal ($d = 0.13$) and nonverbal ($d = 0.19$) for transfer effects given by these authors. Smith et al. (2010) is the source for the exercise effects on working memory; Hedge's $g = 0.56$ is plotted as point *b* in the figure. It is the seventy-first percentile. The meditation memory improvement shown is based on the average of the gains reported by Jensen et al. (2012), Chambers et al. (2008), and Mrazek et al. (2013). This average, Cohen's $d = 0.59$, is plotted in the figure as the seventy-second percentile.

Chapter 7

Page 98

surveys find that forgetting names: Devolder, P. A., & Pressley, M. (1991). Memory complaints in younger and older adults. *Applied Cognitive Psychology*, *5*(5), 443–454.

Page 98

Researcher Lori James studied memory: James, L. E. (2004). Meeting Mr. Farmer versus meeting a farmer: Specific effects of aging on learning proper names. *Psychology and Aging, 19*(3), 515–522. The figure on page 99 shows results from her Experiment 1.

Page 101

some researchers believe specialized neural circuitry: Kanwisher, N., & Yovel, G. (2009). Face perception. In G. G. Berntson & J. T. Cacioppo (Eds.), *Handbook of neuroscience for the behavioral sciences* (Vol. 2., pp. 841–858). Hoboken, NJ: John Wiley & Sons.

Page 101

But if you interact with her: Johnston, R., & Edwards, A. (2009). Familiar and unfamiliar face recognition: A review. *Memory, 17*(5), 577–596.

Page 101

"What you select could be anything": Lorayne, H., & Lucas, J. (1974). *The memory book*, p. 88. Briarcliff Manor, NY: Stein & Day.

Page 102

People differ significantly: Bindemann, M., Avetisyan, M., & Rakow, T. (2012). Who can recognize unfamiliar faces? Individual differences and observer consistency in person identification. *Journal of Experimental Psychology: Applied*, *18*(3), 277–291.

Page 103

memory expert Kenneth Higbee observed: Higbee, K. (2001). *Your memory?: How it works and how to improve it* (2nd ed.), p. 197. New York: Da Capo Press.

Page 104

Seniors appear to be especially vulnerable: Stevens, W. D., Hasher, L., Chiew, K. S., & Grady, C. L. (2008). A neural mechanism underlying memory failure in older adults. *Journal of Neuroscience*, *28*(48), 12820–12824.

Page 105

Mnemonist Scott Hagwood recommends: Hagwood, S. (2007). *Memory power: You can develop a great memory—America's Grand Master shows you how*, p. 107. London: Free Press.

Page 105

research is consistent with his advice: Mangels, J. A., Manzi, A., & Summerfield, C. (2010). The first does the work, but the third time's the charm: The effects of massed repetition on episodic encoding of multimodal face–name associations. *Journal of Cognitive Neuroscience*, *22*(3), 457–473.

Page 105

Psychologist Peter Morris: Morris, P. E., Fritz, C. O., Jackson, L., Nichol, E., & Roberts, E. (2005). Strategies for learning proper names: Expanding retrieval practice, meaning, and imagery. *Applied Cognitive Psychology*, *19*(6), 779–798.

Page 105

When Harry Lorayne amazed audiences: Lorayne was a regular guest on TV variety shows in the 1960s and 1970s, such as those hosted by Jack Parr, Ed Sullivan, and Johnny Carson. His signature feat was to learn the name of everyone in the audience, sometimes hundreds of people. First he was introduced to each individual, and then he would have them all stand. As he identified each by name, they sat down, one after the other, until no one was left standing.

Page 108

Laboratory studies show that both college students: Carney, R. N., & Levin, J. R. (2012). Facing facts: Can the face–name mnemonic strategy accommodate additional factual information? *Journal of Experimental Education*, *80*(4),

386–404. Groninger, L. D., Groninger, D. H., & Stiens, J. (1995). Learning the names of people: The role of image mediators. *Memory*, *3*(2), 147–167. Yesavage, J. A., Rose, T. L., & Bower, G. H. (1983). Interactive imagery and affective judgments improve face–name learning in the elderly. *Journal of Gerontology*, *38*(2), 197–203.

Page 108

In two studies in which students had learned: Both are reported by Morris et al. (2005).

Page 109

Dan Gabor, a business coach: Gabor, D. (2011). *How to start a conversation and make friends* (Revised ed.). New York: Touchstone.

Page 109

Called the "name game": Morris, P. E., & Fritz, C. O. (2000). The name game: Using retrieval practice to improve the learning of names. *Journal of Experimental Psychology: Applied*, *6*(2), 124–129. Morris, P. E., & Fritz, C. O. (2002). The improved name game: Better use of expanding retrieval practice. *Memory*, *10*(4), 259–266.

Page 110

have used it with as many as twenty-five: Morris, P. E., Fritz, C. O., & Buck, S. (2004). The name game: Acceptability, bonus information and group size. *Applied Cognitive Psychology*, *18*(1), 89–104.

Page 110

As Dale Carnegie observed: Carnegie, D. (1936). *How to win friends and influence people*, p. 79. New York: Pocket Books.

Chapter 8

Page 112

By one estimate, over half of the daily memory problems: McDaniel, M. A., & Einstein, G. O. (2007). *Prospective memory: An overview and synthesis of an emerging field*, p. 193. Thousand Oaks, CA: Sage.

Page 112

Although precise numbers aren't known: Weingarten, G. (2009, March 8). Fatal distraction: Forgetting a child in the backseat of a car is a horrifying mistake. But is it a crime? *The Washington Post*. Retrieved from *www.washingtonpost. com/lifestyle/magazine/fatal-distraction-forgetting-a-child-in-thebackseat- of-a-car-is-a-horrifying-mistake-is-it-a-crime/2014/06/16/8ae0fe3a-f580-*

11e3-a3a5-42be35962a52_story.html. Some estimates of heatstroke deaths attributable to parental forgetting are higher than Weingarten's. See *www. kidsandcars.org/heatstroke.html* retrieved on December 27, 2014.

Page 113

"The wealthy do, it turns out": Weingarten (2009).

Page 113

but this is no ordinary memory: McDaniel & Einstein (2007).

Page 113

"slumbers on in the person": Freud, S. (1960). *The psychopathology of everyday life*. (A. Tyson, Trans.), p. 152. New York: W. W. Norton.

Page 114

detected through either top-down or bottom-up processes: This view is known as multiprocess theory in the professional literature (McDaniel & Einstein, 2007).

Page 114

something has to give: Marsh, R. L., Hicks, J. L., & Cook, G. I. (2005). On the relationship between effort toward an ongoing task and cue detection in event-based prospective memory. *Journal of Experimental Psychology: Learning, Memory, and Cognition, 31*(1), 68–75.

Page 114

McDaniel and Einstein believe is our preferred way: McDaniel & Einstein (2007, p. 54).

Page 115

Researchers call this a "focal cue": McDaniel & Einstein (2007, pp. 59–62).

Page 117

psychologist Peter Gollwitzer: Gollwitzer, P. M. (1999). Implementation intentions: Strong effects of simple plans. *American Psychologist, 54*(7), 493–503.

Page 117

how an implementation intention works its magic: McDaniel, M. A., & Scullin, M. K. (2010). Implementation intention encoding does not automatize prospective memory responding. *Memory and Cognition, 38*(2), 221–232. Rummel, J., Einstein, G. O., & Rampey, H. (2012). Implementation-intention encoding in a prospective memory task enhances spontaneous retrieval of intentions. *Memory, 20*(8), 803–817.

Page 117

especially helpful when the cue for the intended action: McDaniel, M. A., Howard, D. C., & Butler, K. M. (2008). Implementation intentions facilitate prospective memory under high attention demands. *Memory and Cognition, 36*(4), 716–724.

Page 118

added benefit for older people: Chasteen, A. L., Park, D. C., & Schwarz, N. (2001). Implementation intentions and facilitation of prospective memory. *Psychological Science, 12*(6), 457–461.

Page 118

The desired action must be a goal you really want: Sheeran, P., Webb, T. L., & Gollwitzer, P. M. (2005). The interplay between goal intentions and implementation intentions. *Personality and Social Psychology Bulletin, 31*(1), 87–98.

Page 118

Some fine points about implementation intentions: Ellis, J. A., & Freeman, J. E. (2008). Ten years on: Realizing delayed intentions. In M. Kliegel, M. A. McDaniel, & G. O. Einstein (Eds.), *Prospective memory: Cognitive, neuroscience, developmental, and applied perspectives* (pp. 1–27). New York: Taylor & Francis Group.

Page 118

helps in many self-control situations: Gollwitzer, P. M., & Sheeran, P. (2006). Implementation intentions and goal achievement: A meta-analysis of effects and processes. In M. P. Zanna (Ed.), *Advances in experimental social psychology* (Vol. 38, pp. 69–119). San Diego, CA: Elsevier Academic Press.

Page 119

it can do this in one of two ways: Kliegel, M., Guynn, M. J., & Zimmer, H. (2007). The role of noticing in prospective memory forgetting. *International Journal of Psychophysiology, 64*(3), 226–232.

Page 119

the cuing stimulus should be in focal attention: McDaniel & Einstein (2007, pp. 59–62).

Page 120

Einstein and McDaniel report that participants: Einstein, G. O., & McDaniel, P. M. A. (2004). *Memory fitness: A guide for successful aging,* p. 135. New Haven, CT.: Yale University Press.

Page 120

create them at the spot: Nowinski, J. L., & Dismukes, R. K. (2005). Effects of ongoing task context and target typicality on prospective memory performance: The importance of associative cueing. *Memory, 13*(6), 649–657.

Page 120

And the more important the task: Kliegel, M., Martin, M., McDaniel, M. A., & Einstein, G. O. (2004). Importance effects on performance in event-based prospective memory tasks. *Memory, 12*(5), 553–561.

Chapter 9

Page 124

Herbert Spitzer carried out a classic study: Spitzer, H. F. (1939). Studies in retention. *Journal of Educational Psychology, 30*(9), 641–656. The figure on page 125 is from his Table 2, time period B1.

Page 125

Their shapes are usually similar: Rubin, D. C., & Wenzel, A. E. (1996). One hundred years of forgetting: A quantitative description of retention. *Psychological Review, 103*(4), 734–760.

Page 125

a powerful, reliable way to enhance memory: Roediger, H. L., Agarwal, P. K., McDaniel, M. A., & McDermott, K. B. (2011). Test-enhanced learning in the classroom: Long-term improvements from quizzing. *Journal of Experimental Psychology: Applied, 17*(4), 382–395.

Page 126

Washington University researchers: Roediger, H. L., & Karpicke, J. D. (2006). Test-enhanced learning: Taking memory tests improves long-term retention. *Psychological Science, 17*(3), 249–255.

Page 127

The results are shown in the bar graph: My graph is based on Figure 1 in Roediger & Karpicke (2006).

Page 127

Multiple-choice tests are a useful way: McDermott, K. B., Agarwal, P. K., D'Antonio, L., Roediger, H. L., & McDaniel, M. A. (2014). Both multiple-choice and short-answer quizzes enhance later exam performance in middle and high school classes. *Journal of Experimental Psychology: Applied, 20*(1),

3–21. But also see McDaniel, M. A., Anderson, J. L., Derbish, M. H., & Morrisette, N. (2007). Testing the testing effect in the classroom. *European Journal of Cognitive Psychology, 19*(4–5), 494–513. Little, J. L., Bjork, E. L., Bjork, R. A., & Angello, G. (2012). Multiple-choice tests exonerated, at least of some charges: Fostering test-induced learning and avoiding test-induced forgetting. *Psychological Science, 23*(11), 1337–1344.

Page 128

the primary studying method: McIntyre, S. H., & Munson, J. M. (2008). Exploring cramming: Student behaviors, beliefs, and learning retention in the Principles of Marketing course. *Journal of Marketing Education, 30*(3), 226–243.

Page 128

the memory boost it provides is short lived: Roediger, H. L., & Karpicke, J. D. (2006). The power of testing memory: Basic research and implications for educational practice. *Perspectives on Psychological Science, 1*(3), 181–210.

Page 129

He calls it "desirable difficulty": Bjork, R. A. (1999). Assessing our own competence: Heuristics and illusions. In D. Gopher & A. Koriat (Eds.), *Attention and performance XVII: Cognitive regulation of performance: Interaction of theory and application* (pp. 435–459). Cambridge, MA: MIT Press.

Page 129

you may not be able to recall it at all: Bahrick, H. P., Hall, L. K., & Baker, M. K. (2013). *Life-span maintenance of knowledge*, p. 226. New York: Psychology Press.

Page 130

Bjork and his colleague: Landauer, T. K., & Bjork, R. A. (1978). Optimum rehearsal patterns and name learning. In M. M. Gruneberg, P. E. Morris, & R. N. Sykes (Eds.), *Practical aspects of memory* (pp. 625–632). New York: Academic Press. Whether expanding retrieval practice leads to more efficient learning than constant spacing is debated by researchers.

Page 130

Professional mnemonists endorse this approach: Buzan, T. (1991). *Use your perfect memory: Dramatic new techniques for improving your memory* (3rd ed.), p. 82. New York: Plume. Hagwood, S. (2007). *Memory power: You can develop a great memory—America's Grand Master shows you how*, p. 72. New York: Free Press. Lorayne, H., & Lucas, J. (1974). *The memory book*, p. 32. Briarcliff Manor, NY: Stein & Day. O'Brien, D. (2000). *Learn to remember?: Practical techniques and exercises to improve your memory*, p. 81. San Francisco: Chronicle Books.

Page 131

students report they rarely use it: Karpicke, J. D., Butler, A. C., & Roediger, H. L. (2009). Metacognitive strategies in student learning: Do students practise retrieval when they study on their own? *Memory, 17*(4), 471–479.

Page 131

memory researcher Jennifer McCabe: McCabe, J. (2011). Metacognitive awareness of learning strategies in undergraduates. *Memory and Cognition, 39*(3), 462–476.

Page 132

an "illusion of competence" after restudying: Bjork (1999).

Page 132

Researcher Mark McDaniel and his collaborators: McDaniel, M. A., Howard, D. C., & Einstein, G. O. (2009). The read-recite-review study strategy: Effective and portable. *Psychological Science, 20*(4), 516–522.

Page 133

the most popular student self-testing strategy: Wissman, K. T., Rawson, K. A., & Pyc, M. A. (2012). How and when do students use flashcards? *Memory, 20*(6), 568–579.

Page 133

the evidence doesn't support this concern: Carpenter, S. K. (2012). Testing enhances the transfer of learning. *Current Directions in Psychological Science, 21*(5), 279–283.

Page 133

taught a group of students how to classify birds: Jacoby, L. L., Wahlheim, C. N., & Coane, J. H. (2010). Test-enhanced learning of natural concepts: Effects on recognition memory, classification, and metacognition. *Journal of Experimental Psychology: Learning, Memory, and Cognition, 36*(6), 1441–1451.

Page 134

The SCRR Method: Similar to the cue word method in Bellezza, F. (1982). *Improve your memory skills.* Englewood Cliffs, NJ: Prentice-Hall.

Page 134

there is a memory benefit to delaying: Butler, A. C., Karpicke, J. D., & Roediger, H. L. (2007). The effect of type and timing of feedback on learning from multiple-choice tests. *Journal of Experimental Psychology: Applied, 13*(4), 273–281.

Page 135

three perfect passes may be better: Karpicke, J. D., & Roediger, H. L. (2007). Repeated retrieval during learning is the key to long-term retention. *Journal of Memory and Language, 57*(2), 151–162.

Page 135

five additional rehearsals spaced a week apart: Rawson, K. A., & Dunlosky, J. (2011). Optimizing schedules of retrieval practice for durable and efficient learning: How much is enough? *Journal of Experimental Psychology: General, 140*(3), 283–302.

Page 136

a visual approach called "mind mapping": Buzan, T., & Buzan, B. (1996). *The mind map book: How to use radiant thinking to maximize your brain's untapped potential.* New York: Plume.

Page 137

this repository of long-lasting information: Bahrick, H. P. (1984). Semantic memory content in permastore: Fifty years of memory for Spanish learned in school. *Journal of Experimental Psychology: General, 113*(1), 1–29. The figure on page 137 is the average of Spanish–English and English–Spanish tests given in his Table 6 and expressed relative to the scores of his Group 0 who took the test immediately after completing their last Spanish course.

Page 138

permastore memories vary in strength. Memories with intermediate strength will sometimes be able to be recalled and other times not, as discussed by Bahrick, Hall, & Baker (2013).

Page 138

long-lasting memories have been found: Bahrick, H. P., Bahrick, P. O., & Wittlinger, R. P. (1975). Fifty years of memory for names and faces: A cross-sectional approach. *Journal of Experimental Psychology: General, 104*(1), 54–75. Bahrick, H. P., & Hall, L. K. (1991). Lifetime maintenance of high school mathematics content. *Journal of Experimental Psychology: General, 120*(1), 20–33. Schmidt, H. G., Peeck, V. H., Paas, F., & van Breukelen, G. J. P. (2000). Remembering the street names of one's childhood neighbourhood: A study of very long-term retention. *Memory, 8*(1), 37–49.

Page 138

memory for high school classmates: Bahrick, Bahrick, & Wittlinger (1975).

Chapter 10

Page 141

a place in the *Guinness Book of World Records:* Retrieved June 25, 2014, from *www.guinnessworldrecords.com/world-records/1/most-pi-places-memorised*. Other mnemonists have claimed to have broken Chao Lu's record, but the claims have not been accepted by the Guinness organization at this time.

Page 141

Chao Lu was inspired: Estimates of the value of pi were proposed many times, even as far back as 1650 B.C. Zu Chongzhi earned special note because he computed a particularly accurate version to seven decimal digits in A.D. 480. It remained the best estimate of pi for 800 years. The quotation from Chao Lu was retrieved on June 25, 2014, from *www.newsgd.com/culture/peopleandlife/200611280032.htm*.

Page 141

Chao Lu planned to recite 90,000 digits: Retrieved June 25, 2014, from *www. pi-world-ranking-list.com/lists/details/luchaointerview.html*. His preparation is described by Hu, Y., Ericsson, K. A., Yang, D., & Lu, C. (2009). Superior self-paced memorization of digits in spite of a normal digit span: The structure of a memorist's skill. *Journal of Experimental Psychology: Learning, Memory, and Cognition, 35*(6), 1426–1442.

Page 141

he cooperated with Chinese and American psychologists: Hu, Ericsson, Yang, & Lu (2009), and Hu, Y., & Ericsson, K. A. (2012). Memorization and recall of very long lists accounted for within the Long-Term Working Memory framework. *Cognitive Psychology, 64*(4), 235–266.

Page 144

The Number-Shape System: Most of my number–shape examples come from Buzan, T. (1991). *Use your perfect memory: Dramatic new techniques for improving your memory* (3rd ed.), p. 52. New York: Plume; and O'Brien, D. (2005). *How to develop a brilliant memory week by week*, p. 42. London: Duncan Baird.

Page 147

Allan Paivio traced its early form: Paivio, A. (1971). *Imagery and verbal processes*, p. 168. New York: Holt, Rinehart & Winston.

Page 147

To get a feel for the code: The answers: 95, 72, 68, 55.

Page 147

Now try your hand at finding words: Some possibilities: 41, rod, or rat or radio; 19, tub or dope or teepee; 47, rock or rug or rag; 35, mule or mail or mole.

Page 147
"a beautiful naked blonde": Lorayne, H., & Lucas, J. (1974). *The memory book,* p. 105. Briarcliff Manor, NY: Stein & Day.

Page 150
Researchers have found that the major system: Patton, G. W., D'Agaro, W. R., & Gaudette, M. D. (1991). The effect of subject-generated and experimenter-supplied code words on the phonetic mnemonic system. *Applied Cognitive Psychology, 5*(2), 135–148.

Page 150
Mnemonist and memory researcher Kenneth Higbee: Higbee, K. L. (1997). Novices, apprentices, and mnemonists: Acquiring expertise with the phonetic mnemonic. *Applied Cognitive Psychology, 11*(2), 147–161.

Page 150
Francis Bellezza, a researcher at Ohio University: Bellezza, F. S., Six, L. S., & Phillips, D. S. (1992). A mnemonic for remembering long strings of digits. *Bulletin of the Psychonomic Society, 30*(4), 271–274.

Page 151
Ben Pridmore, a top British mnemonist, remembers numbers: Pridmore's system is described at *http://mnemotechnics.org/wiki/Ben_System,* retrieved on June 25, 2014. He was the overall winner at the 2008 World Memory Championship based on ten events. Memorizing 1,800 numbers in an hour is currently his best performance in that event.

Page 151
Say O'Brien wants to remember: O'Brien calls his person–action approach the "Dominic System" and describes it in O'Brien (2005).

Page 153
The approach Chao Lu took: Hu & Ericsson (2012); also see Hu et al. (2009).

Page 153
Satan may relish coffee pie: Memory trainer Francis Fauvel-Gouraud seems to be the originator of this mnemonic. Fauvel-Gouraud, F. (1845). *Phreno-mnemotechny: Or, The art of memory,* p. 120. New York: Wiley and Putnam. Retrieved from *books.google.com/books*.

Page 153
the set of code words I use: My code words were largely derived from those presented by Higbee, K. (2001). *Your memory: How it works and how to improve it* (2nd ed.), pp. 219–222. New York: Da Capo Press; and Bellezza, F. (1982).

Improve your memory skills, pp. 119–123. Englewood Cliffs, NJ: Prentice-Hall. The newer online word generators for the Major System are even better sources.

Chapter 11

Page 155
the Starbucks acronym: Duhigg, C. (2012). *The power of habit: Why we do what we do in life and business*, p. 145. New York: Random House.

Page 157
These perceptual skill are every bit as important: Causer, J., Janelle, C. M., Vickers, J. N., & Williams, A. M. (2004). Perceptual expertise: What can be retained? (pp. 306–324). In N. J. Hodges & A. M. Williams (Eds.), *Skill acquisition in sport*. New York: Routledge.

Page 157
Psychologists describe the behavior as automatic: Moors, A., & De Houwer, J. (2006). Automaticity: A theoretical and conceptual analysis. *Psychological Bulletin, 132*(2), 297–326.

Page 158
Some skills are more about mental operations: Rosenbaum, D. A., Carlson, R. A., & Gilmore, R. O. (2001). Acquisition of intellectual and perceptual-motor skills. *Annual Review of Psychology, 52*, 453–470.

Page 159
has studied top performers: Ericsson, K. A., & Lehmann, A. C. (1996). Expert and exceptional performance: Evidence of maximal adaptation to task constraints. *Annual Review of Psychology, 47*, 273–305.

Page 160
Ericsson called this "deliberate practice": Ericsson, K. A. (2006). The influence of experience and deliberate practice on the development of superior expert performance. In K. A. Ericsson, N. Charness, P. J. Feltovich, & R. R. Hoffman (Eds.), *The Cambridge handbook of expertise and expert performance* (pp. 683–703). New York: Cambridge University Press.

Page 160
An important part of deliberate practice is problem solving: Ericsson, K. A. (2003). The acquisition of expert performance as problem solving: Construction and modification of mediating mechanisms through deliberate practice.

In J. E. Davidson & R. J. Sternberg (Eds.), *The psychology of problem solving* (pp. 31–83). New York: Cambridge University Press.

Page 161
elite achievers typically invest ten years: Ericsson, K. A., Krampe, R. T., & Tesch-Römer, C. (1993). The role of deliberate practice in the acquisition of expert performance. *Psychological Review, 100*(3), 363–406.

Page 162
Here is a successful Olympian: Orlick, T., & Partington, J. (1988). Mental links to excellence. *The Sport Psychologist, 2*(2), 112.

Page 162
At the 2014 Sochi Winter Games: Clarey, C. (2014, February 22). Olympians use imagery as mental training. *The New York Times*. Retrieved from *www. nytimes.com/2014/02/23/sports/olympics/olympians-use-imagery-as-mental-training.html*.

Page 162
Earlier studies of Olympic contenders: Murphy, S. M. (1994). Imagery interventions in sport. *Medicine and Science in Sports and Exercise, 26*(4), 486–494. Ungerleider, S., & Golding, J. M. (1991). Mental practice among Olympic athletes. *Perceptual and Motor Skills, 72*(3, Pt. 1), 1007–1017.

Page 162
a well-researched principle in psychology: Driskell, J. E., Copper, C., & Moran, A. (1994). Does mental practice enhance performance? *Journal of Applied Psychology, 79*(4), 481–492. Suinn, R. M. (1997). Mental practice in sport psychology: Where have we been, where do we go? *Clinical Psychology: Science and Practice, 4*(3), 189–207. Schuster, C., Hilfiker, R., Amft, O., Scheidhauer, A., Andrews, B., Butler, J., et al. (2011). Best practice for motor imagery: A systematic literature review on motor imagery training elements in five different disciplines. *BMC Medicine, 9*(75), 1–35.

Page 162
works best when your imagined performance: Smith, D., Wright, C., Allsopp, A., & Westhead, H. (2007). It's all in the mind: PETTLEP-based imagery and sports performance. *Journal of Applied Sport Psychology, 19*(1), 80–92.

Page 163
I recommend that you prepare a written script: For suggestions on preparing scripts, see Williams, S. E., Cooley, S. J., Newell, E., Weibull, F., & Cumming,

J. (2013). Seeing the difference: Developing effective imagery scripts for athletes. *Journal of Sport Psychology in Action, 4*(2), 109–121.

Page 164

keep in mind that it is itself a skill: Gould, D., Voelker, D. K., Damarjian, N., & Greenleaf, C. (2014). Imagery training for peak performance. In J. L. Van Raalte & B. W. Brewer (Eds.), *Exploring sport and exercise psychology* (3rd ed.), pp. 55–82. Washington, DC: American Psychological Association.

Page 164

British researcher Ian Glendon: Glendon, A. I., McKenna, S. P., Hunt, K., & Blaylock, S. S. (1988). Variables affecting cardiopulmonary resuscitation skill decay. *Journal of Occupational Psychology, 61*(3), 243–255.

Page 165

a loss of competence over time: Sabol, A., & Wisher, R. A. (2001). Retention and reacquisition of military skills. *Military Operations Research, 6*(N1), 59–80. Arthur, W. J., Bennett, W. J., Stanush, P. L., & McNelly, T. L. (1998). Factors that influence skill decay and retention: A quantitative review and analysis. *Human Performance, 11*(1), 57–101.

Page 165

The Red Cross recommends: Retrieved June 25, 2014 from *www.redcrossrefresher.com/q/first-aid-cpr-and-aed/choices.*

Page 165

The great pianist Ignacy Paderewski: The quote is from Francis, C. (2009). *Wisdom well said*, p. 331. El Prado, NM: Levine Mesa Press.

Page 165

A typical F-15 pilot: Levy, C. P. (2006). *A comparison study of F-15C fighter squadron ready aircrew program flying hour scheduling vs. the Rand Corporation's flying hour scheduling linear program (AFIT/IOA/ENS/06-04).* Wright-Patterson Air Force Base, OH: Air Force Institute of Technology.

Chapter 12

Page 170

"I am thirty-four years old": Parker, E. S., Cahill, L., & McGaugh, J. L. (2006). A case of unusual autobiographical remembering. *Neurocase, 12*(1), 35.

Page 171

write down the date that Easter fell on: She made one mistake listing the twenty-four Easters by giving a date that was two days off. Two years later, she was asked without warning to repeat the task. This time she was correct on all the dates and gave very similar memories for each of the days. When she was shown her earlier responses, she immediately pointed out the incorrect date (Parker et al., 2006).

Page 171

McGaugh and his team carefully studied many: LePort, A. K. R., Mattfeld, A. T., Dickinson-Anson, H., Fallon, J. H., Stark, C. E. L., Kruggel, F., Cahill, L., & McGaugh, J. L. (2012). Behavioral and neuroanatomical investigation of Highly Superior Autobiographical Memory (HSAM). *Neurobiology of Learning and Memory, 98*(1), 78–92.

Page 172

Gillian Cohen and Dorothy Faulkner: Cohen, G., & Faulkner, D. (1988). Life span changes in autobiographical memory. In M. M. Gruneberg, P. E. Morris, & R. N. Sykes (Eds.), *Practical aspects of memory: Current research and issues, Vol. 1: Memory in everyday life.* (pp. 277–282). Oxford, U.K.: John Wiley & Sons. Additional details are provided by Williams, H. L., Conway, M. A., & Cohen, G. (2008). Autobiographical memory. In G. Cohen & M. A. Conway (Eds.), *Memory in the real world* (3rd ed.), pp. 21–90. New York: Psychology Press.

Page 172

David Pillemer and his colleagues: Pillemer, D. B., Goldsmith, L. R., Panter, A. T., & White, S. H. (1988). Very long-term memories of the first year in college. *Journal of Experimental Psychology: Learning, Memory, and Cognition, 14*(4), 709–715. The figure on page 173 is based on their Figure 1.

Page 174

"I was woken up by a thundering noise": Berntsen, D., & Thomsen, D. K. (2005). Personal memories for remote historical events: Accuracy and clarity of flashbulb memories related to World War II. *Journal of Experimental Psychology: General, 134*(2), 257.

Page 174

This was a flashbulb event worldwide: Curci, A., & Luminet, O. (2006). Follow-up of a cross-national comparison on flashbulb and event memory for the September 11th attacks. *Memory, 14*(3), 329–344.

Page 174

"Another curious aspect of medieval justice": Bishop, M. (2001). *The Middle Ages*, p. 217. Boston: Mariner Books.

Page 175

by hitting one another: Bishop (2001, p. 116).

Page 175

Emotional memories are usually relatively accurate: Reisberg, D., & Heuer, F. (2004). Memory for emotional events. In D. Reisberg & P. Hertel (Eds.), *Memory and emotion* (pp. 3–41). New York: Oxford University Press.

Page 175

Lia Kvavilashvili and her colleagues: Kvavilashvili, L., Mirani, J., Schlagman, S., Foley, K., & Kornbrot, D. E. (2009). Consistency of flashbulb memories of September 11 over long delays: Implications for consolidation and wrong time slice hypotheses. *Journal of Memory and Language, 61*(4), 556–572.

Page 175

an impressive body of research shows: Talarico, J. M., & Rubin, D. C. (2009). Flashbulb memories result from ordinary memory processes and extraordinary event characteristics. In O. Luminet & A. Curci (Eds.), *Flashbulb memories: New issues and new perspectives* (pp. 79–97). New York: Psychology Press.

Page 175

This "bump" is illustrated in the graph: Redrawn from Figure 2 in Rubin, D. C. (2002). Autobiographical memory across the lifespan. In P. Graf & N. Onta (Eds.), *Lifespan development of human memory* (pp. 159–184). Cambridge, MA: MIT Press.

Page 176

The bump is probably due to: Rubin (2002, pp. 173–174).

Page 177

it's that their memories don't last: Bauer, P. (2012). The life I once remembered: The waxing and waning of early memories. In D. Berntsen & D. C. Rubin (Eds.), *Understanding autobiographical memory* (pp. 205–225). New York: Cambridge University Press.

Page 177

Part of the reason is brain development: Bauer, P. J. (2007). *Remembering the times of our lives: Memory in infancy and beyond*. Mahwah, NJ: Lawrence Erlbaum.

Page 177

Children have to learn how: Nelson, K., & Fivush, R. (2004). The emergence of autobiographical memory: A social cultural developmental theory. *Psychological Review, 111*(2), 486–511.

Page 177

By the time they are eight or nine: Bauer (2012, p. 208).

Page 177
The life stories they are beginning to formulate: Habermas, T., & Bluck, S. (2000). Getting a life: The emergence of the life story in adolescence. *Psychological Bulletin, 126*(5), 748–769.

Page 177
Researchers call collections of memories: Thomsen, D. K. (2009). There is more to life stories than memories. *Memory, 17*(4), 445–457.

Page 178
Martin Conway, a prominent researcher: Conway, M. A., & Pleydell-Pearce, C. W. (2000). The construction of autobiographical memories in the self-memory system. *Psychological Review, 107*(2), 261–288.

Page 179
Four scientific articles have now appeared: Parker et al. (2006). LePort et al. (2012). Ally, B. A., Hussey, E. P., & Donahue, M. J. (2013). A case of hyperthymesia: Rethinking the role of the amygdala in autobiographical memory. *Neurocase, 19*(2), 166–181. Patihis, L., Frenda, S. J., LePort, A. K. R., Petersen, N., Nichols, R. M., Stark, C. E. L., McGaugh, J. L., & Loftus, E. F. (2013). False memories in highly superior autobiographical memory individuals. *Proceedings of the National Academy of Sciences, 110*(52), 20947–20952. Also see comments on a case in Baddeley, A. D. (2012). Reflections on autobiographical memory. In D. Berntsen & D. C. Rubin (Eds.), *Understanding autobiographical memory* (pp. 81–82). New York: Cambridge University Press.

Page 179
Jill Price recalls that December 19, 1980: Price, J. (2008). *The woman who can't forget: The extraordinary story of living with the most remarkable memory known to science—A memoir*, pp. 27–28. New York: Free Press.

Page 179
a marked tendency toward obsessiveness: LePort et al. (2012).

Page 180
One woman, Louise Owen: Finkelstein, S. (Producer). (2010, December 19). Endless memory. Parts 1 and 2. *60 Minutes*. New York: CBS.

Page 180
In between these extremes: Cornoldi, C., De Beni, R., & Helstrup, T. (2007). Memory sensitivity in autobiographical memory. In S. Magnussen & T. Helstrup (Eds.), *Everyday memory*. (pp. 183–199). New York: Routledge. Merriam, S. B. (1993). Butler's life review: How universal is it? *International Journal of Aging and Human Development, 37*(3), 163–175.

Page 180

women engage in autobiographical remembering: Grysman, A., & Hudson, J. A. (2013). Gender differences in autobiographical memory: Developmental and methodological considerations. *Developmental Review, 33*(3), 239–272.

Page 181

not all autobiographical remembering is healthy: O'Rourke, N., Cappeliez, P., & Claxton, A. (2011). Functions of reminiscence and the psychological well-being of young-old and older adults over time. *Aging and Mental Health, 15*(2), 272–281.

Page 181

Constructive reminiscing: Westerhof, G. J., & Bohlmeijer, E. T. (2014). Celebrating fifty years of research and applications in reminiscence and life review: State of the art and new directions. *Journal of Aging Studies, 29,* 107–114.

Page 181

"In my sophomore year": Pillemer, D. B. (2001). Momentous events and the life story. *Review of General Psychology, 5*(2), 130.

Page 181

"It was embarrassing, not making that team": Pillemer (2001, p. 127).

Page 181

majority of autobiographical memories will be positive: Walker, W. R., Skowronski, J. J., & Thompson, C. P. (2003). Life is pleasant—and memory helps to keep it that way! *Review of General Psychology, 7*(2), 203–210.

Page 181

under the guidance of a psychotherapist: Hallford, D., & Mellor, D. (2013). Reminiscence-based therapies for depression: Should they be used only with older adults? *Clinical Psychology: Science and Practice, 20*(4), 452–468.

Page 182

the three-step process: Henner, M. (2012). *Total memory makeover: Uncover your past, take charge of your future,* pp. 3–5. New York: Gallery Books.

Page 183

Marilu Henner suggests identifying life-story chapters: Henner (2012, pp. 140–143).

Page 183

In one study of middle-aged people: Thomsen, D. K., Olesen, M. H., Schnieber,

A., & Tønnesvang, J. (2014). The emotional content of life stories: Positivity bias and relation to personality. *Cognition and Emotion*, *28*(2), 260–277.

Page 184
Studies have identified jewelry: Habermas, T., & Paha, C. (2002). Souvenirs and other personal objects: Reminding of past events and significant others in the transition to university. In J. D. Webster & B. K. Haight (Eds.), *Critical advances in reminiscence work: From theory to application* (pp. 123–139). New York: Springer.

Page 184
they are avid collectors: LePort et al. (2012).

Page 184
Memory expert Dominic O'Brien: O'Brien, D. (2000). *Learn to remember: Practical techniques and exercises to improve your memory*, p. 144. San Francisco: Chronicle Books.

Page 184
The way you picture memories: Rice, H. J. (2010). Seeing where we're at: A review of visual perspective and memory retrieval. In J. H. Mace (Ed.), *The act of remembering: Toward an understanding of how we recall the past* (pp. 228–258). West Sussex, UK: Wiley-Blackwell.

Page 185
"I see myself dancing at a party": Berntsen, D., & Rubin, D. C. (2006). Emotion and vantage point in autobiographical memory. *Cognition and Emotion*, *20*(8), 1193.

Page 185
Forcing a memory: Vella, N. C., & Moulds, M. L. (2014). The impact of shifting vantage perspective when recalling and imagining positive events. *Memory*, *22*(3), 256–264.

Page 185
Henner identified four ways: Henner (2012, pp. 87–90).

Page 187
"I know that part of the reason": Henner (2012, p. 24).

Page 187
Habits are a special kind of memory: Graybiel, A. M. (2008). Habits, rituals, and the evaluative brain. *Annual Review of Neuroscience*, *31*, 359–387. Wood,

W., & Neal, D. T. (2007). A new look at habits and the habit-goal interface. *Psychological Review, 114*(4), 843–863.

Page 187

"autobiographical state of mind": Henner (2012, p. 177).

Page 187

Habits are established by repeating: The key operation is pairing the cue and the behavior over and over. The positive outcome motivates the sequence so that it occurs often enough to form the habit. Once the habit is firmly in place, the positive outcome is believed to be unnecessary (Wood & Neal, 2007).

Page 189

"try to think of bad memories": Henner (2012, pp. 38–39).

Page 189

In one study, students undertook to develop: Lally, P., van Jaarsveld, C. H. M., Potts, H. W. W., & Wardle, J. (2010). How are habits formed: Modelling habit formation in the real world. *European Journal of Social Psychology, 40*(6), 998–1009.

Chapter 13

Page 191

you needn't worry that you might confuse: Massen, C., & Vaterrodt-Plünnecke, B. (2006). The role of proactive interference in mnemonic techniques. *Memory, 14*(2), 189–196.

Page 191

The peg word strategy excels in two areas: These two key functions of mnemonics are discussed by Bellezza, F. S. (1996). Mnemonic methods to enhance storage and retrieval. In E. L. Bjork & R. A. Bjork (Eds.), *Memory* (pp. 345–380). San Diego, CA: Academic Press.

Page 192

peg words get high marks: Worthen, J. B., & Hunt, R. R. (2011). *Mnemonology: Mnemonics for the 21st century.* New York: Psychology Press.

Page 193

Other well-known acronyms: Evans, R. L. (2007). *Every good boy deserves fudge: The book of mnemonic devices.* New York: Perigee.

Page 194

"Poorly Canned Sausages": Anonymous. (1972). *A dictionary of mnemonics,* p. 27. London: Eyre Methuen.

Page 194
Planning on serious partying?: Anonymous. (1972, p. 26). Follow this advice at your own risk!

Page 195
memory researcher David Rubin pointed out: Rubin, D. C. (1995). *Memory in oral traditions: The cognitive psychology of epic, ballads, and counting-out rhymes.* New York: Oxford University Press.

Page 195
memorize the entire *Aeneid*: Carruthers, M. (2008). *The book of memory: A study of memory in medieval culture* (2nd ed.), p. 21. New York: Cambridge University Press.

Page 196
committed the entire *Quran* to memory: Luo, M. (2006, August 16). Memorizing the way to heaven, verse by verse. *The New York Times.* Retrieved from *www.nytimes.com/2006/08/16/nyregion/16koran.html.*

Page 196
"Starting with envelope/airplane": Lorayne, H. (2007). *Ageless memory: Simple secrets for keeping your brain young,* p. 41. New York: Black Dog & Leventhal.

Page 197
On the mnemonic scorecard: Bellezza (1996).

Page 199
In one study, college students: Bower, G. H., & Clark, M. C. (1969). Narrative stories as mediators for serial learning. *Psychonomic Science, 14*(4), 181–182. Also see Worthen & Hunt (2011, pp. 72–73).

Page 199
tested after periods longer than a few days: Boltwood, C. E., & Blick, K. A. (1970). The delineation and application of three mnemonic techniques. *Psychonomic Science, 20*(6), 339–341.

Page 199
shown to work with older adults: Drevenstedt, J., & Bellezza, F. S. (1993). Memory for self-generated narration in the elderly. *Psychology and Aging, 8*(2), 187–196.

Chapter 14

Page 202
Reports say he seldom took notes: Leibovich, M. (2005, January 5). Pressure

cooker. *The Washington Post.* Retrieved from *www.washingtonpost.com/wp-dyn/content/article/2006/03/28/AR2006032800445.html.*

Page 203

A 2005 *Washington Post* story: Leibovich (2005).

Page 204

Simonides, also known as "the honey tongued": Yates, F. A. (1996). *The art of memory,* p. 42. London: Pimlico.

Page 205

There were no chapter titles: Small, J. P. (1997). *Wax tablets of the mind: Cognitive studies of memory and literacy in classical antiquity,* pp. 11–25. London: Routledge.

Page 206

Memory scholar Mary Carruthers believes: Carruthers, M. (1998). *The craft of thought: Meditation, rhetoric, and the making of images, 400–1200,* p. 9. New York: Cambridge University Press.

Page 206

The great Catholic theologian Thomas Aquinas: Yates (1966, pp. 81–90) describes how Thomas restated the principles of the Method of Loci for the medieval period. Memory skill as a step on the path to moral perfection is discussed by Carruthers, M. (2008). *The book of memory: A study of memory in medieval culture* (2nd ed.), p. 88. New York: Cambridge University Press. Thomas's own memory skill is described by Carruthers (2008, pp. 3–9).

Page 207

"to roam across a hundred thousand memory images": Spence, J. D. (1985). *The memory palace of Matteo Ricci,* p. 9. New York: Penguin Books.

Page 207

It is a personification of "grammar": This is Plate 7a in Yates (1966). Other depictions of grammar for mnemonic purposes were also in play at this time as variations on the Method of Loci. Interesting examples of "towers of grammar" are examined by Mittelberg, I. (2002). The visual memory of grammar: Iconographical and metaphorical insights. Retrieved July 2, 2014, from *www.metaphorik.de/en/journal/02/visual-memory-grammar-iconographical-and-metaphorical-insights.html.*

Page 208

Rhetoric, on the other hand: Spence (1985, p. 8).

Page 209
"I told them they should write down": Spence (1985, p. 139).

Page 210
They just did not find Ricci's memory techniques helpful: Ricci's instructions also suffered from some cultural disconnects with Chinese readers as discussed by Hsia, R. P. (2010). *A Jesuit in the forbidden city: Matteo Ricci 1552–1610*. Oxford, UK: Oxford University Press.

Page 210
Contemporary studies show: Custers, E. J. F. M. (2010). Long-term retention of basic science knowledge: A review study. *Advances in Health Sciences Education, 15*(1), 109–128.

Page 211
forces were in play that led to its decline: Yates (1966). Rossi, P. (2000). *Logic and the art of memory: The quest for a universal language* (S. Clucas, Trans.). Chicago: University of Chicago Press.

Page 213
When I take care of one of these tasks: Once I have no more use for a memory cue at a specific location, it just goes away. Andrew Card experienced the same when he took a memory cue to his disposal. It is an interesting phenomenon researchers have studied as "directed forgetting." Baddeley, A., Eysenck, M. W., & Anderson, M. C. (2009). *Memory,* pp. 221–224. New York: Psychology Press.

Page 215
My approach is similar to one: My list generally follows Lorayne, H., & Lucas, J. (1974). *The memory book*, p. 137. Briarcliff Manor, NY: Stein & Day. These mnemonists use a peg word system to remember the deck of cards, not a memory palace. I find the memory palace is easier to manage.

Page 216
use more complex coding systems: Foer, J. (2011). *Moonwalking with Einstein: The art and science of remembering everything*, pp. 165–167. New York: Penguin Press. O'Brien, D. (2005). *How to develop a brilliant memory week by week*, pp. 149–151. London: Duncan Baird. O'Brien also explains how he set up a memory palace to hold 2,808 cards.

Page 218
medieval monks believed: Carruthers (1998, pp. 173–174).

Chapter 15

Page 221

Carol Dweck, a researcher at Stanford: Dweck, C. (2006). *Mindset: The new psychology of success.* New York: Random House.

Page 221

a study by Dweck and Claudia Mueller: Mueller, C. M., & Dweck, C. S. (1998). Praise for intelligence can undermine children's motivation and performance. *Journal of Personality and Social Psychology, 75*(1), 33–52.

Page 222

compares the number of problems children solved: My figure shows data averaged across Studies 1, 3, and 5 from Mueller & Dweck (1998) as presented in her Figure 2.

Page 223

A recent review summarized: Burnette, J. L., O'Boyle, E. H., VanEpps, E. M., Pollack, J. M., & Finkel, E. J. (2013). Mind-sets matter: A meta-analytic review of implicit theories and self-regulation. *Psychological Bulletin, 139*(3), 655–701.

Page 224

the widespread stereotype that advancing age: Chasteen, A. L., Kang, S. A., Remedios, J. D. (2012). Aging and stereotype threat: Development, process and interventions. In M. Inzlicht & T. Schmader (Eds.), *Stereotype threat: Theory, process and applications* (pp. 202–216). New York: Oxford University Press. Hess, T. M., & Emery, L. (2012). Memory in context: The impact of age-related goals on performance. In M. Naveh-Benjamin & N. Ohta (Eds.), *Memory and aging: Current issues and future directions* (pp. 183–214). New York: Psychology Press.

Page 224

conducted by Catherine Haslam: Haslam, C., Morton, T. A., Haslam, S. A., Varnes, L., Graham, R., & Gamaz, L. (2012). "When the age is in, the wit is out": Age-related self-categorization and deficit expectations reduce performance on clinical tests used in dementia assessment. *Psychology and Aging, 27*(3), 778–784.

Page 225

the impact of stereotypes on cognitive performance: Inzlicht, M., & Schmader, T. (2012). *Stereotype threat: Theory, process, and application.* New York: Oxford University Press.

Page 225

Those who thought of themselves as old: Stereotype effects arise in several ways. Sometimes they can be similar to "choking" under pressure, but with the elderly it appears more often to be a loss of motivation. Hess, T. M., Hinson, J. T., & Hodges, E. A. (2009). Moderators of and mechanisms underlying stereotype threat effects on older adults' memory performance. *Experimental Aging Research, 35*(2), 153–177.

Page 226

encouraged to adopt a growth mindset: Hong, Y., Coleman, J., Chan, G., Wong, R. Y. M., Chiu, C., et al. (2004). Predicting intergroup bias: The interactive effects of implicit theory and social identity. *Personality and Social Psychology Bulletin, 30*(8), 1035–1047.

Page 226

Researchers Jason Plaks and Allison Chasteen: Plaks, J. E., & Chasteen, A. L. (2013). Entity versus incremental theories predict older adults' memory performance. *Psychology and Aging, 28*(4), 948–957.

Page 226

can help anyone who has low expectations: A paper discussing this point from the perspective of neurologically impaired individuals is Kit, K. A., Tuokko, H. A., & Mateer, C. A. (2008). A review of the stereotype threat literature and its application in a neurological population. *Neuropsychology Review, 18*(2), 132–148.

Page 227

Carol Dweck has identified two different forms: Dweck, C. S. (1986). Motivational processes affecting learning. *American Psychologist, 41*(10), 1040–1048. Also see Hastings, E. C., & West, R. L. (2011). Goal orientation and self-efficacy in relation to memory in adulthood. *Aging, Neuropsychology, and Cognition, 18*(4), 471–493. Stout, J. G., & Dasgupta, N. (2013). Mastering one's destiny: Mastery goals promote challenge and success despite social identity threat. *Personality and Social Psychology Bulletin, 39*(6), 748–762.

Index

About the Author

Robert Madigan, PhD, is Professor Emeritus of Psychology at the University of Alaska Anchorage, where he was an award-winning instructor. Dr. Madigan has taught memory classes in college and community settings for more than thirty years. He lives in Anchorage with his wife.